TANGLED TONGUE

Tangled Tongue

LIVING WITH A STUTTER

JOCK A. CARLISLE

University of Toronto Press
Toronto Buffalo London

© University of Toronto Press 1985
Toronto Buffalo London
Printed in the U.S.A.

ISBN 0-8020-2558-7 (cloth)
ISBN 0-8020-6577-5 (paper)

Canadian Cataloguing in Publication Data
Carlisle, Jock A. (Jock Alan), 1924–
    Tangled tongue: living with a stutter
    Bibliography: p.
    Includes index.
    ISBN 0-8020-2558-7 (bound). – ISBN 0-8020-6577-5 (pbk.)
    1. Carlisle, Jock A. (Jock Alan), 1924–
    2. Stuttering. 3. Stuttering – Treatment. I. Title.
    RC424.C37 1985   616.85′54   C85-098689-3

This book is dedicated to my much loved wife, Joan,
who has helped me pick up the pieces of my life so many
times.

Publication of this book has been assisted by the
Ontario Arts Council under its block grant program.

Contents

Acknowledgments

This book could not have been written without the encouragement and help of my wife, Joan, who typed so many drafts that she more than earned her IBM word processor.

I shall always be grateful to the speech rehabilitation team led by Susan Carrol-Thomas at the Royal Ottawa Hospital's Regional Rehabilitation Centre, particularly to Ann Meltzer, Anne Godden, Carol Dixon, and Vicky Inns for their compassion, perceptiveness, and unswerving dedication. Dr Norman Ward of Ottawa deserves special thanks for his wise counsel and for placing his finger gently on so many tender truths.

I wish to thank all the people who reviewed the manuscript and made helpful, constructive criticisms, particularly Professor Einer Boberg, Susan Carrol-Thomas, and Ann Meltzer. The comments and encouragement of the 'dean' of Speech Pathology, Professor Charles Van Riper, made the struggle of revising the book worth while.

My thanks also go to my literary agent, Joanne Kellock of Edmonton, whose eagle eye and sense of balance saved me from drowning my readers in a deep well of words.

I wish to acknowledge the many store clerks, waitresses, hotel receptionists, car-hire clerks, airline booking clerks, telephone operators, and others who unwittingly played important roles as guinea pigs in testing various speech techniques and observing the responses.

Ann Dewar of Edinburgh University, Mike Hughes of St John, New Brunswick, and Findlay, Irvine Ltd., of Penicuik, Scotland, kindly provided information about the Edinburgh viii Acknowledgments

Masker. I also wish to express my appreciation to those speech pathologists in North America, Europe, South Africa, Australia, and Japan who provided the data about stuttering and speech centres. The scientific attachés of the different embassies were most helpful in making the overseas contacts.

My thanks go to Virgil Duff and the other members of the editorial and marketing staff of the University of Toronto Press for their encouragement and advice. Their help was invaluable.

For permission to refer in the text to other published works, I am indebted to: the National Easter Seals Society and to Professor Oliver Bloodstein, author of the masterly *A Handbook on Stuttering* (1969, 1981); Pergamon Press (Oxford) for material from H.E. Beech and F. Fransella, *Research and Experiment in Stuttering*; Doubleday (New York) for material from Richard M. Restak, *The Brain: the Last Frontier*; Faber and Faber (London), Random House Inc. (New York), and Alfred A. Knopf, Inc. (New York) for the quotations from W.H. Auden and C. Isherwood's *The Ascent of F6*; William Morrow Co. Inc. (New York) for material from *Peter's Quotations*; and Prentice-Hall, Inc. (Englewood Cliffs, NJ) and Professor Charles Van Riper for material from *Speech Correction: Principles and Methods*.

Warm thanks go to the many patients of the Royal Ottawa Hospital Regional Rehabilitation Centre for their friendship, support, good humour, and courage in spite of the difficulties they face every day. They were the best possible companions on a difficult voyage.

I remember our therapy sessions as times of affection, laughter, adventure, and determination. They will never be forgotten. Particular thanks go to Bob and Dolly Smith who, besides brightening the day for every person they met, gave so freely of their time and experiences.

Last but not least, I wish to thank my three daughters – Kate, Sara, and Susan – for not being aware of the tangle in my tongue while they were growing up.

Preface

Six people patiently waited to order their burgers, french fries, and Cokes at Harvey's in Pembroke, Ontario. As my turn approached I felt the familiar tightening of my stomach muscles and adjusted my mind to handle the ordeal ahead. My wife, Joan, hovered in the background, encouraging but nervous.

I soon found myself facing the smiling, uniformed girl at her microphone, and said, 'Two chicken sandwiches, please, one with sauce, one without sauce, one portion of french fries, and two coffees. We'll eat them here.' The girl smiled, repeated the order over the intercom, took my money, and wished me a nice day. 'Next please!'

Joan joined me at the counter while the food was being prepared and, with a big smile and eyes flashing with pleasure, said, 'Terrific! You did it! Did you see her face and watch her eyes? They didn't change! It worked!' It was the best fast-food lunch we had ever eaten. This type of scene takes place millions of times every day in Canada and the United States, but for me it was a unique experience.

I had had difficulty speaking for about fifty-five years and, although at times I was more or less fluent, there were some situations I could never handle. Ordering food in a stand-up situation was one of them. By about the third word I always stuttered and went into a block of prolonged silence while the person behind the counter became embarrassed, nervous, or even hostile. Sometimes I couldn't start at all, and then eyes would glaze as the order-taker waited. When someone tittered in the background it took a tremendous effort to control both my feelings and my temper and to get my speech back on course. I always got there in the end, but ill feelings would crackle on both sides of the counter.

This type of experience happens nearly every time anybody with a severe stutter goes into a store, a restaurant, or any public place where he has to ask for something.

On that particular day I was trying out an electronic device, called the Edinburgh Masker, which stops you from hearing your own speech and makes speaking easier for some people.[1] The masker does not work equally well for everybody. Even when it works it isn't foolproof, and you need to think carefully about the technique when you speak. Nevertheless, on this day the snares and pitfalls in the sentences needed to order the sandwiches melted away, I slid slowly through the words, and the girl's face did not change to an expression of anxiety or hostility. I entered an unfamiliar world where people did not automatically react badly whenever I opened my mouth.

I tested the instrument in many situations for a week or more and found it surprisingly effective. Since then the masker has had varied effects on my stutter; but in general it has made life easier. I can seek telephone assistance without causing the operator to become abusive or insolent, ask for merchandise in stores, and chat to people in the street, all without the need for a tight rein on my feelings and articulation.

During fifty years of speech therapy I have often heard other patients say, 'If only I could speak perfectly for one day – just one bloody day – I'm sure I could control my stutter.' They have a point. Since the day I ordered the chicken sandwiches my speech has been much more controlled, with or without the masker.

Many years ago I stood on top of a mountain leaning on my ice axe. Looking at the sparkling-white, windswept world through my tinted snow goggles, I made a promise that if I could learn to control my speech, even for a short time, I would help other people who stutter by writing a book to explain their problems to the rest of the world. This book fulfils that promise.

My purpose in writing was to cast some light on the mystery surrounding the causes of stuttering; the kind of people who stutter, and the difficulties they face every day; the ways stuttering can be treated; and the responses of society to this strange, erratic way of speaking.

Although the book deals with a disability, above all it is about people – the kind of people who face life with a handicap that society finds hard to understand and accept.

Most writing about disabilities views the patient from the outside, but in this case the viewpoint is that of the patient looking outward at life.

The focus is stuttering, but many of the problems described relate to other disabilities, particularly those that interfere with communication. Deaf people may recognize parallels with their own situations.

People who stutter can be fluent one minute and completely speechless the next. The intermittence and apparent unpredictability of the speech make listeners nervous. The average person may know, more or less, how to deal with a blind or deaf person, a paraplegic, an amputee, or someone who is mentally handicapped; but very few people know what to do when faced by a stutterer. Do you help the guy begin his word? Do you look at him or look away as he struggles to speak? Do you smile encouragingly or sit there like a stuffed dummy? Most people look away, fidget, and think of ways to escape; or, if they happen to be holding a cup of coffee, stir it as though their lives depend upon it. Many just flee in alarm as the stutterer battles his way to the next word. Few know what to do, and uncertainty breeds fear with its attendant tension, rudeness, hostility, and anger. To make matters worse stutterers' own attitudes vary – some welcome help and others do not. All stutterers welcome a little patience.

Stutterers can exhibit such bizarre tics and grimaces when they try to speak that people think they are mad, or at best wildly eccentric. Some people feel, incorrectly, that anybody who loses control of his speech is mentally impaired and treat him accordingly. They may also wonder why someone will speak fluently on some occasions and stutter on others.

Stuttering interferes with the attribute that sets human beings apart from all the other animals – the aptitude for verbal communication. Other mammals – whales, for example – communicate by signals, but only humans have the gift of expressing complex thoughts in spoken words. Speech is the basis of our culture. The inability to communicate fluently affects every moment of a stutterer's life and tends to push him or her outside society.

W.H. Auden, in his dramatic poem *The Ascent of F6*, writes about 'the girl imprisoned in the tower of a stutter.' I prefer to think of people who stutter as living in a *glass* tower. The glass wall is placed there by society. Stutterers can see people and hear them, but cannot reach out and touch them physically or mentally. They would gladly walk out and mingle with people, but every time they speak the transparent, impenetrable wall closes around them.

It is hoped that this book will help to shatter or at least crack this glass wall and remove misconceptions about the disability. The book is not a scientific, in-depth study of the origins of stuttering and how to cure it, although these subjects are discussed in some detail. There are plenty of publications on the psychology, physiology, and treatment of stuttering; but few discuss a stutterer's relationships with other people.

I am not a speech therapist or a psychiatrist but, after fifty-five years of stuttering and fifty years of therapy, I am familiar with most forms of treatment and can claim to be an authority on *my* stutter. A hen may not be an expert on the physiology of eggs, but she knows better than anybody else what it feels like to lay an egg.

Although this book is not an autobiography, many of the incidents described were experienced or seen by me. Others I heard of from responsible people or read about in books written by reliable authors. Wherever possible the incidents are described unchanged, but in cases where participants would be embarrassed I have modified the circumstances, location, and personal descriptions to prevent identification.

Often, people who stutter have an acute appreciation of the absurd and face their problems with remarkable courage and good humour. Nevertheless, although they can laugh at the ludicrous situations they encounter, they take strong exception to being ridiculed or patronized. Some parts of this book describe funny situations, but this does not mean that stuttering is just an amusing aberration to be taken lightly. Far from it. Living with a stutter – dealing with its social effects every day – is no laughing matter.

Throughout the book the word 'stuttering' is used. This is the North American term for 'stammering' (British), *'begaiement'* (French), *'balbuzie'* (Italian), *'stottern'* (German), *'tartamudez'* (Spanish), and *'gagueira'* (Portuguese).[2] The disability has also been called 'spasmophemia,' 'laloneurosis,' and 'balbuties' in the scientific literature.[3]

Some writers group stuttering and cluttering[4] into the single category of 'clutter-stuttering.' In this text stuttering, with its complex, unclear origins, is considered separately from cluttering, a different type of disorder, which is apparently caused by neurological abnormality. It is recognized that some stutterers also clutter and that the borderline between the two disabilities is not clear.

Most speech therapists are women and they are referred to as 'she.' The masculine third person 'he' is used for stutterers, but no disrespect is meant to women, lib. or non-lib. Four out of five people with stutters are male, and a surfeit of 'he or she's' would be tedious. Ugly words such as 'chairperson' and 'salesperson' are widely used and I could have written 'stutterperson,' but that would have been absurd. So 'he' it is, and I'll just have to take my lumps. May the Creator, wherever she is, forgive me.

TANGLED TONGUE

'I wouldst thou couldst stammer, that thou mightst pour this concealed man out of thy mouth, as wine comes out of a narrow-mouthed bottle; either too much at once, or none at all.'

William Shakespeare

ONE

What is a stutter?

'A man is hid under his tongue.'

Ali-Ibn-Abi-Talib (seventh century)

During the 1950s a speech therapist asked me to write down a definition of a stutter, and I thought it would be easy. I wrote down all the key terms – 'blocking,' 'repetition,' 'lack of rhythm,' and so on – and had nearly finished my masterpiece when he leaned over my shoulder and said, 'While you're at it, tell me how a stutter differs from untidy normal speech and from the other speech disorders you've encountered.' After an hour all I had was a page full of notes, but my mentor said, 'Not to worry! I don't know either. I just thought you might come up with a bright idea!'

Everybody knows what a severe stutter looks and sounds like with its tics, blocks, and repetitions, but inarticulate people with normal speech also frequently pause and repeat. When one patient was asked to describe his stutter briefly he replied, 'Downright embarrassing! A darned nuisance!' The point was that he blocked and repeated to such an extent that his hesitations inconvenienced him, made him feel anxious and uncomfortable, and handicapped him in daily life. It is these sorts of consequences that distinguish a stutter from normal disfluency.

This is still a little vague, and the United States Health Service was cautious when it wrote: 'Stuttering remains an enigma while illustrating the type of disorder which does not have a clear organic cause or a clearly habitual basis.'[1] A cop-out, yes, but an honest cop-out.

Enigma or not, it is very clear to me what I am writing about. Most experts agree that, in general, a stutter is the interruption of the flow of speech by hesitations, prolongation of sounds, avoidance of difficult words, struggles to speak, and blockages sufficient to cause anxiety and impair verbal communication. Other symptoms may or may not be associated with the stutter. These include low self-esteem, grimacing, stamping the foot, clenching the hands, twisting the fingers, protruding the tongue, looking away, closing the eyes, and contorting the body in the enormous effort to move from one word to the next.

Speech disorders that are not stutters involve some of these symptoms. People suffering from aphasia following a stroke may have speech blockages in addition to difficulty in choosing the right words to form syntax that makes sense. They don't stutter. The hasty, sloppy, stumbling, jerky speech of a clutterer in some ways resembles a stutter, but is quite different.

People who stutter often detach themselves completely when they freeze into a prolonged block. While the listener and the stutterer wait for the locked lips or tongue to release for communication to continue, the stutterer may go into a kind of trance. His articulatory muscles seem to be carved from stone and, without therapy to provide him with a key to his lock, he is helpless and in danger of (literally) running out of air. The strange part is the depth of the detachment. While a stutterer is frozen in a block, people can slam doors, shout 'Fire,' or tell him that he has won a lottery, with no response whatsoever. I used to plan the next day's activities and remind myself to pay bills and complete my income tax return during long blocks, while my audience patiently or impatiently waited for speech to continue. A major speech block is hard to describe, but many stutterers feel completely out of touch as they wait for release.

It is difficult for the layman to differentiate between normal lack of fluency and the hesitations and repetitions of some stutterers. If you listen to any radio talk-show or analyse any political speech, you will notice that many speakers, besides mangling English grammar and syntax, include a remarkable number of hesitations in every spoken sentence. I remember hearing an opera singer interviewed on the radio. She paused, repeated, blocked, and said 'um,' 'ah,' and 'er' to such an extent that it was hard to understand her. She was not a stutterer, or a clutterer, nor did she have aphasia. She was just inarticulate. It is hoped that she sang better than she talked.

Even with children it is difficult to tell the difference between normal childish disfluency and the hesitations and repetitions that develop into a full-blown stutter. A parent may be unaware that the child has a stutter, or may think that the child is starting to stutter when he is only normally hesitant. Some children use highly abnormal repetitions of individual sounds, as many as forty, at an age of four or less. It seems likely that these children will develop stutters.

Lacking any clear definition, I shall describe the kind of stutter I am going to write about – my kind. My speech was, and still is to some extent, impaired by intermittent, unpredictable difficulty in progressing from one sound to the other, with repetition, stumbling, and debilitating blocking – sometimes lasting as long as thirty seconds – leading to a complete breakdown of verbal communication. In particular, the blocking type of stutter can be a major handicap to communication and social involvement.

A stutter can vary so much from day to day, or even from hour to hour, that people tend to underestimate its importance. It is not such an obvious, continual handicap as blindness, deafness, or paralysis of the limbs, all of which have received considerable attention from the medical profession and sympathy from the public. A person who stutters severely can usually manage his life fairly well and learns to cope with the fear, despair, humiliation, and frustration that accompany him every time he talks to strangers and sees their change of expression, asks for a meal and encounters rudeness, or tries to make a telephone call and meets impatience or worse.

A stutter is not just inarticulacy; it includes a whole syndrome of effects that feed back to the person who stutters and make his speech worse. Rebuffs and rejection are as much a part of stuttering as the speech blockages and interruptions. People who react badly to stuttering are not usually deliberately unkind. They respond to their fear that they cannot cope with the unfamiliar situation and tend to copy the behaviour of others toward people with noticeable disabilities. Stuttering is not part of their usual experience.

A small boy and his father watched a group of adults tormenting a beautiful green snake in a slippery plastic bucket. Tiring of the sport, the tormentors tipped the snake out and laughingly crushed its head underfoot. When the perplexed boy asked why they tormented and killed the harmless reptile, his father replied, 'A snake is just not part of their world.'

TWO

Questions people are afraid to ask – and things they shouldn't say

'He who asks a question is a fool for five minutes; he who does not ask a question is a fool for ever.'

Chinese Proverb

People who stutter can sometimes be prickly about their impediment, particularly when they are not willing to admit even to themselves that they have a handicap. Others will discuss their disability freely. When you first meet a stutterer you don't know what kind of person he is. If you ask him a question about his speech you may get short shrift with 'Mind your own business,' or you may launch your companion on his favourite topic – his stutter.

If you manage to start a conversation, you may want to ask questions about stuttering, but feel diffident about doing so in case you intrude upon the stutterer's privacy. People meeting a person with a stutter for the first time tend to be as wary in their conversation as though picking their way through a verbal minefield. The purpose of this chapter is to defuse some of the mines and correct some misconceptions.

Do you help a stutterer with his words, offer advice, or look away?

This trilogy of questions strikes at the core of the difficulties a stutterer encounters when dealing with people in stores,

restaurants, and other social situations. People who meet a
stutterer don't know what to do.

I accompanied a young man with a severe stutter into a
store to try out his newly learned speech techniques by ordering some cigarettes. On the second word he blocked badly.
Instead of using the speech techniques, he panicked and tried
to push through the word with quivering, pursed lips. The
eyes of the woman behind the counter went blank. She
shrugged, walked away to serve another customer, and never
returned.

The stutterer, without his cigarettes, was in a cold fury, but
after he'd calmed down we tried again at another store. He
blocked again, but the pleasant girl behind the counter gave
him her full attention, maintained eye contact without staring, and patiently waited the few seconds he needed to collect
himself and apply his techniques. There was no problem.

In the first situation the response of the ill-mannered, impatient woman was bad and made the stutter worse. The second case demonstrated how a little patience and pleasant,
helpful feedback helped the stutterer recover from his block.
The way you respond to a stutterer will greatly affect his
speech. Don't look away or leave him as soon as you find a
plausible excuse. Just act with normal good manners. Most
stutterers dislike it intensely when people switch them off and
walk away to spare their own feelings.

Whether you should help a stutterer complete a blocked
word is best answered by, 'When in doubt, don't.' Some people who stutter severely welcome help, but if they are under-
going therapy their therapist won't thank you for finishing
words or sentences. If your urge to help is overwhelming, ask
the stutterer, 'Would you like me to complete your difficult
words or not?' He'll probably say no, but at least you'll both
know where you stand.

The majority of stutterers find it difficult when somebody
ends their words and sentences for them because the comple-
tion is usually not what they wanted to say, which means that
they need to start all over again. Some irritating people are
compulsive sentence-finishers, even with people who have
normal speech. One stutterer spoke longingly of consigning
sentence-finishers to a syntactical hell where small devils in-

terrupted their victims in the middle of each sentence and completed it with words meaning the complete opposite of what they wanted to say. Anybody can be forgiven for wanting to throttle a person who, as you struggle to say 'I went for my holiday in G___' fills in with the word 'Glasgow' when you really wanted to say exotic 'Guadeloupe.'

Stutterers may be pestered by well-meaning people asking tactless questions and offering bad advice. Winston Churchill is to be admired as a wartime leader, but he is the bane of stutterers' lives as far as speech is concerned. At social occasions over-familiar strangers may say challengingly, 'Churchill cured his stutter. Why can't you?' The implication is that your failure indicates a lack of moral fibre. I don't know how bad Churchill's stutter was, and I am not sure that he cured it. His articulacy in political oratory was amazing, but it is said that he still stuttered in conversation. I would like to lay Churchill and his stutter to rest a second time, and hope that his ghost will cease to haunt the stutterers of the world.

Another statement guaranteed to raise a stutterer's hackles is, 'I once stuttered very badly, but I worked at it and look at me now!' (Yes, look at him – the tactless so-and-so!) A variant of this is, 'I had a friend (aunt, uncle, girl-friend, mistress) who stuttered but he (she) overcame it by sheer determination!' These statements are usually followed by suggestions that you relax, take a deep breath, clench your left fist, say 'er' before every word, tap your foot, or have faith in yourself. These unofficial experts frequently end by saying, 'You can cure your stutter if you *really* want to,' implying that since you still have an impediment you are a weak-kneed jellyfish.

Then there are the purveyors of gloom and doom who urge you to be realistic and face facts. They say that they've read a great deal about stuttering and to them it is clear that you'll never get any better. One of these individuals tactfully left on my desk a large tome by a man with a German name so long I looked for the verb at the end. The heavy-faced author, pictured with a crew-cut, bushy moustache, black tails, and pin-stripe pants, ran a speech clinic somewhere in Bavaria where stutterers were bludgeoned into fluency by talking as they rhythmically marched up and down and clapped their hands.

When they failed to be fluent, they were consigned to guilt-ridden psychological purgatory. On the last page – which was flagged for my attention – the expert declared that if you stuttered after the age of forty the problem would get worse and worse and cast you into an inarticulate, lonely old age – unless you went to old crew-cut's clinic and paid his huge fees.

People who offer unsolicited advice may be well intentioned, but they can be a trial, like those people who knock on your door and give you religious tracts and a homily about how to achieve salvation. They seem to assume that you've never given the matter a moment's thought.

The person who stutters wants your full attention. For him, speaking is hard work, and nothing is more exasperating than someone who, as the stutterer tries to disentangle his speech, carries on a side-conversation with other people. One of my daughters used to do this. She still lives, which speaks well for my self-control.

Most people who stutter communicate remarkably well using their abnormally disfluent speech, plus the body language through which much is communicated even by people with normal speech. Words are only one way of conveying information. Albert Mehrabian found that only about 7 per cent of communication involves words. The rest consists of non-verbal vocal or paralinguistic cues (38 per cent) and facial expressions (55 per cent).[1] Non-verbal communication came before complex speech in the evolution of man. Even today babies learn to communicate long before they can talk.

In recent years, sociologists and anthropologists have shown increasing interest in the science of kinesics, which is concerned with the implications of patterns of behaviour in non-verbal communication. This new science caught the interest of the public under the 'body language' label as part of the wave of pop-psychology that swept the Western world during the 1970s.[2]

If a person who stutters doesn't get your attention, he cannot use his non-verbal skills, and this may be one of the reasons he finds it so hard to use the telephone.

What do you do when speaking to a stutterer? Be patient, don't look away, don't fill in words or end sentences, don't offer unsolicited advice. Just act with ordinary good manners. It's not very difficult.

What kind of people stutter?

During the 1970s I participated in group therapy sessions as both a patient and a hospital volunteer at the Royal Ottawa Hospital in Ottawa. On Thursday nights adult patients with stutters assembled in a room and discussed their problems and progress. It was a great challenge to speak in a controlled manner to twenty or more people under the watchful eyes of the therapists. Most of us were nervous, so I made a list of the age, sex, ethnic origin, and occupations of the patients in the room to calm my feelings.

The stutterers' ages ranged from about eighteen to sixty-four, and about a fifth of the group were girls. There were a few students, a teacher, a forester, a labourer, a scientist, four civil servants, a girl with a beaded headband and buckskins, a storekeeper, a pig farmer, an auto-mechanic, a fireman, a man and a woman in the restaurant business, a soldier, a recreation specialist, a political scientist, a statistician, a truck driver, a building contractor, and a novice priest from a seminary who had trouble saying grace.

The patients were Canadians with Chinese, Greek, Jewish, Italian, French, and British backgrounds. Many of them were doing well in their jobs, but had encountered difficulties while speaking to customers, making telephone calls, addressing meetings, or ordering cattle feed. They were there to ease the tension and anxiety in their lives by learning to control their erratic speech.

Some had already had a great deal of therapy, and they maintained reasonable fluency as they spoke to the group using the speech techniques they had been taught. Others were obviously tense. Their throat muscles involuntarily quivered, their lips trembled, and their faces twitched nervously as they slowly described their progress, prolonging every word and striving to keep in touch with their speech and maintain eye contact with the audience. There were people who were confident, insecure, shy, humorous, solemn, extroverted, introverted, aggressive, and timid. People of all races, professions, and characters have stutters. It is a myth that all people who stutter are shy, unsociable, moronic, and introverted.

Each person responds to having a stutter in his own way depending on his personality. There are braggarts and buffoons who wave their stutters in public like a flag, just as there are timid people driven into solitude and despair by their handicap. Some are totally crushed by the stress of trying to speak; but most cope from day to day and arrange their lives so that their stuttering interferes as little as possible.

The people in the group mixed remarkably well considering the differences in education, interest, occupation, age, and ethnic origin. Some were easier to get along with than others, but most were warm, friendly, and intelligent. Although they had all been stressed and battered by the daily need to cope with their disfluent speech, the majority were remarkably unsoured by their experiences. I enjoyed their company, even when the therapy frayed my nerves as I tried to do mundane but seemingly impossible tasks like making a collect telephone call.

The group had a boisterous sense of humour, and meetings were great fun, with bright repartee and kindly teasing punctuated by gusts of laughter. The patients trusted each other with their feelings, and their respect for the therapists was obvious. There was so little unkindness, bitchiness, selfishness, self-pity, and hostility that I looked forward to the sessions as a relief from the competitive work situation. They restored my wilting confidence in humanity. People who stutter have a great deal to offer if others have the patience and the good manners to listen to them.

About 1 per cent of school children in North America, Europe, and Australia stutter. The impediment seems to be less common in the United States (about 0.7 per cent) than in Europe (about 1.1 per cent); it is relatively common in Poland (1.7 per cent).

The data generally refer to school children rather than adults because young people are captive participants in school surveys. The figures reflect an equilibrium because some children recover from their impediment while others develop it.

Inventories of children and adults who either have stutters or at some time stuttered and recovered have given results far higher than 1 per cent. Oliver Bloodstein gives rates ranging from about 5 to 15 per cent and averaging about 10 per cent.[3] In North America about 2.5 million people are known to stutter; this number takes no account of people who successfully hide their stutters and adults who don't report their handicap or request therapy. The true figure is probably much higher.

A stutterer like myself, who has had many years of therapy, can spot another stutterer as soon as he opens his mouth, even when he is fluent. I can identify those who use speech techniques to keep fluent and spot those who hide their stutter by word substitution, changes in accent, and shifts in role. It becomes a sixth sense.

I unobtrusively surveyed two research establishments where I worked; 3 per cent of the staff of a laboratory in Britain had stutters, and 6 per cent of a research institute in Canada. Some of the stutterers who didn't have prolonged speech blockages seemed to be unconcerned about their problem. Others hid their disfluency nearly perfectly. Nevertheless, they stuttered – no doubt about it.

Do some types of people stutter more than others? Yes, more boys stutter than girls. The ratio of boys with stutters to girls varies between 2:1 and 6:1, but on average about four boys stutter for every girl with the same problem. This preponderance of male stutterers has caused a great deal of speculation, and some authorities feel it reflects the relatively slow speech development of boys and the congenital vulnerability of the male constitution compared with females. Others feel that boys encounter more competition and frustration in speaking than girls, while another school of thought feels that parents react differently to normal hesitations in a boy's speech than in a girl's.[4] It may be that girls just speak more easily than boys. At the age of five, all my minuscule girl-friends had the gift of gab. In a mixed group of children the only way for me to get a word in edgeways was to bat a girl with my teddy bear.

Whether people who stutter are more or less intelligent than people without stutters has been the subject of much debate. Many people feel that because a person cannot control his speech he must be stupid or mad. There are many stories about stutterers who, because they grimaced in their struggles to speak, were certified insane by ill-informed physicians and confined in mental institutions for many years. Even today there is a tendency to look upon people with severe stutters as mentally impaired. It is true that some people with severe mental handicaps stutter, but some of them also have deficiencies of vision and hearing. Nobody links these disabilities with mental impairment.

Stutterers and their families and friends often counter these unfounded accusations by saying that people with stutters are *more* intelligent than others. They refer to the many famous and intelligent people in history who had the disability. There is no doubt that some exceptionally bright people stutter, but the scientific evidence about the relationship between stuttering and intelligence is conflicting. The trouble is that stuttering can be confused with other speech disabilities such as cluttering, and even with normal inarticulacy. The main tool used to measure intelligence is the IQ test, which has been misused and misunderstood ever since it was invented. There does not seem to be any simple way of ranking human intelligence within the normal range. The IQ takes little account of a person's innate abilities to use intuitive thought and to adapt, both of which have been and still are vital in mankind's mental evolution. A person with a stutter may have such low self-esteem that it affects his performance in any test situation. Some people have an aversion to tests in general, and a person with perfectly normal intelligence may get a low test score.

The IQ test was designed by a Frenchman, Alfred Binet, in 1908, for a specific, limited purpose: to identify children with learning disabilities or mild retardation who needed special education. The IQ was modified by W. Stern in 1912 and in its final form is a person's mental age divided by his chronological age and multiplied by 100. The test consists of a series of graded questions, of increasing complexity, that average children of different ages can answer. It simply assesses mental age.

The test is useful for identifying definite mental abnormalities. Unfortunately, like many other good ideas, the IQ has been misused, particularly in the education systems of North America, where educators have tended to use it blindly as an index of relative intelligence of normal children, labelling a child as stupid or bright for the rest of his or her scholastic life. There are people with low IQ scores who are intelligent, effective citizens; and there are people with genius IQs who are ineffective ninnies. In the next century, the IQ test as an index of relative intelligence of normal people will probably join craniometry in the rag-bag of quaint and misused scientific ideas.

For the record, children with stutters at schools and speech clinics in the United States have IQs ranging from low (54) to very high (162) and averaging 95–100, which is similar to the average for the population as a whole. A few studies imply that stutterers are slightly more common among people with lower IQ scores, but these results have not withstood close scrutiny because of problems of sampling and lack of suitable experimental controls. There is some evidence that stuttering students at universities are more intelligent than the average student, but in general stutterers seem to be neither brighter nor more stupid than the average Joe on the street.[5]

The Clan of the Tangled Tongue includes the prophet Moses and the philosophers Demosthenes and Aristotle. Emperors and kings (Emperor Claudius of Rome, and kings Charles I and George VI of England) and statesmen (Thomas Jefferson, Winston Churchill, and Aneuran Bevan) stuttered, and some well-known scientists (Isaac Newton, Erasmus Darwin, and Charles Darwin) and authors (Virgil, Aesop, Charles Lamb, Nevil Shute, Arnold Bennett, and Somerset Maugham) had trouble with their speech. Some public figures, film stars, television personalities, and musicians (Lorne Green, Eric Roberts, Marilyn Monroe, Gary Moore, Jack Paar, Annie Glenn, and Mel Tillis) managed to cope in public in spite of their blocks and hesitations, and many professors of speech pathology, psychiatrists, and speech therapists have been troubled by tangled tongues, particularly the eminent Wendell Johnson, Charles Van Riper, Joseph Sheehan, Hugo Gregory, and Einer Boberg.

The list is endless. All these people rose to prominence by great effort and courage in spite of their stuttering. Some may feel that the challenging barriers imposed by the disability provided the impetus that drove them to the top.

Twins tend to be more prone to develop stutters than others, and estimates range from a nearly normal 1.9 per cent[6] to as high as 13 per cent.[7] Although this has genetic implications, the slowness of maturation and competitive pressure between the individuals in a twin pair have been suggested as possible causes of the high incidence of stuttering in twins.[8]

Unless you stutter yourself you can't tell if a person stutters just by looking at him, or even listening to him. A person can chat to you for an hour or so, and you may have no idea that he stutters. One attractive girl in her twenties had been married for several years. She worked in a government office and requested therapy because the stress of concealing her stutter from her employers was affecting her health. Her husband had no idea that she stuttered. When the therapists persuaded her to stutter openly to relieve the tension of concealment it was quite a surprise to her family. People with moderately severe stutters can get away with hiding it for years – but they pay a price.

The simple answer to the question about what kind of people stutter is that all kinds of people stutter. The impediment can affect kings as well as paupers.

Why don't you stutter when you sing, whisper, or speak in unison?

It is true that many stutterers can sing, whisper, or speak in unison fluently, but the degree of fluency tends to vary from person to person, and their speech can let them down when they least expect it. The reasons for fluency in these situations are far from clear.

At the age of eleven, when I had a moderate but not debilitating stutter, I had the misfortune to possess an exceptionally clear, well-pitched, soprano voice, which led to my being shanghaied into performing as soloist at many local concerts. I objected to singing solo carols and traditional songs in cavernous churches and dusty school halls. I loathed wearing a white robe and a starched collar that rubbed my neck raw. But the teachers were bigger than I was, so there was no use protesting.

I became blasé about the whole thing. It was all a bit of a bore, but I had done it before and could do it again. All I had to do was go on stage, sing, and go home for baked beans on toast.

My nemesis caught up with me in Blackpool, a town in northwestern England, where I was to sing 'Strawberry Fair.' With feelings of resignation and boredom, I stood on a wooden dais on a large dusty stage. The curtain went up and there was a burst of applause from a sea of faces before me. To my horror I found I was alone on the stage of the Blackpool Opera House being grilled to a clinker by bright lights. Instead of the usual scattering of parents and teachers, I faced a huge, packed auditorium.

The orchestra struck up the introduction, I opened my mouth, and there was dead silence. Not a squeak. The violins quaveringly petered out, the conductor rapped for my attention, and we tried again. Not a chirrup. I blocked completely on my easiest word, 'As.' The audience began to shuffle, and I fled, but the teachers bullied me back on to the platform. There I stood, plain mad and bloody-minded, sang like an angry lark, stumped scowling off the stage, and bashed a bigger boy in the wings who dared to giggle.

Singing can increase fluency, but it can also catch you bending. People often ask, 'Why don't you sing every time you speak?' (Tra, la, la.) I curb my inner reply of, 'Don't be daft!' and politely say that it just doesn't work. Singing for me is not communication; it seems to involve different mechanisms from those I use when I express thoughts and feelings in speech.

Unless one sings dirty lyrics in the wrong company or indulges in political satire in a totalitarian state, the content of a song doesn't have potentially dire consequences for the singer. Children and adults are well aware that words have power for good or bad and evoke responses and consequences. In common with most people with the same impediment, I am more likely to stutter the higher the message content of the words.

It seems possible that when a stutterer is singing, the fact that he is playing another role helps his fluency. This effect of role on speech is skimmed over by many textbooks on stuttering, although it is known that some adolescent stutterers have difficulty perceiving their own life roles.[9] I know several apparently fluent people who hide their stutters completely by changing their accents when they get into blocks. One man switches so swiftly from unaccented English to broad Scottish, to cockney, to Welsh, or to American that it leaves me bewildered and wondering which person he really is. He keeps perfectly fluent by switching his roles, but it is exhausting to listen to him.

One stutterer, who later became a therapist, completely controlled a moderate stutter at the age of twenty-five by participating in amateur theatricals. He was fluent when he played roles other than himself, and this improved his speech off the stage. It makes me wonder which role he played away from the theatre to maintain his fluency.

Some pundits say that stutterers can sing because their breathing is controlled, or because they are more concerned with voice pitch and volume than words, or because of a change in role, but these are all guesses.

Stutterers whisper fairly fluently as a rule. I could always talk *sotto voce* in churches and libraries where I was supposed to be silent. (Even so, the fluent whisper can collapse.)

Why whispering helps fluency is another mystery. The common explanations involving theories about speech concealment, role-playing, and distraction don't bear close examination. There may be something to the explanation that when the stutterer's lower speech frequencies are blanked out so that he can't hear them he is usually more fluent. These low frequencies seem to interfere with speech.[10] and whisperers don't use low frequencies, so there is less risk of speech interference. But the answer to the question of why stutterers can whisper fluently probably lies in the interaction of many factors.

The fact that stutterers can read poems in class in unison with other people but not alone is puzzling. I was fluent in unison, but would block completely when I tried to read aloud on my own, and this led to misunderstandings. Several teachers said, 'You see! You *can* speak fluently! You just don't *try*,' and penalties usually followed. This intermittent fluency leads to the belief that the stutterer can easily choose not to stutter, so that people may penalize him for selecting the wrong option. Absurd though this is, a stuttering child at school who shows that he can be fluent can make himself a bed of nails.

I used to think that I could speak in unison because I could hardly hear my voice, but this theory was scuttled by the fact that when I wanted to make a fluent tape recording of a speech or scientific paper, I could do so if my wife read in unison in a whisper so low that the microphone did not pick it up. Reading in unison made me feel more relaxed about my speech. Possibly, sharing the responsibility of communicating and having someone to fall back on when I got into trouble helped my fluency. Possibly, the presence of a distraction accounted for it. All of these theories hold about enough water to float a matchstick. The fact is that nobody really knows the answer.

When my speech was exceptionally bad it helped to read slowly in unison with somebody, but it was at best a crutch. No one can go around speaking in unison all the time unless he happens to be a Siamese twin with a co-operative partner, and then he has other problems.

People who stutter tend to be more fluent when they shadow another person's speech, and one form of therapy was based on this fact. The stutterer produces a running copy of somebody else's speech. I used to spend hours shadowing radio announcers, but unfortunately the beneficial effects ceased immediately when I spoke to anybody else. The shadowing may have temporarily improved my fluency because I was concentrating on another person's voice and had my attention distracted from the stutter, or because I was not communicating and did not need to synchronize my thoughts with my speech.

Distracting a stutterer's attention away from his speech often improves fluency and some therapies are based on this fact. During World War II there were moments when my thoughts were so distracted by the possibility of imminent extinction that I became noisily and vehemently fluent.

Do you stutter when you've had a few drinks?

Yes, I do! I stutter in my sleep, under narcotics, or filled to the gills with good Scotch whiskey – preferably pure malt. Several drinks make some stutterers fluent and others completely speechless.

I've experimented with many speech-improvement techniques, but the whiskey trials were the most fun. At the time, I was a student and had a bad cold, so I decided to kill two birds with one stone by combining the Scottish Bowler Hat Treatment for colds with research on the effects of alcohol on my stutter.

The Bowler Hat Treatment is an old and respected remedy whereby you go to bed with a bottle of good malt whiskey and a bowler hat. You hang the bowler hat at the foot of the bed and leisurely sip the whiskey until you see two, or preferably three, bowler hats. By this time you can be sure that either the cold is cured or you can't feel it. I tried this technique in my lodgings and, although the whiskey did wonders for my cold, it rendered me speechless. That does not mean that I was silent, because my landlady complained about my bawdy songs in the night and nearly showed me the door.

More seriously, alcohol relaxes people and affects their co-ordination – that's why we have breathalyser tests. Relaxation helps some stutterers to control their speech, but alcohol interferes with the co-ordination of most stutterers' systems and makes their speech worse. Theoretically, enough alcohol to relax the stutterer but not sufficient to interfere appreciably with his co-ordination should improve his fluency. The effects will vary from person to person and there's no harm in doing a few enjoyable experiments.

Do you stutter on your own?

I can read aloud and speak on my own fairly fluently if I am careful to keep my rate of speech below eighty words a minute, to prolong words, and to approach the first sounds of words gently. Nevertheless stress enters my speech after a while, and I have to watch techniques very carefully indeed or I start to block. Even talking to a dog or cat can increase the blocks, and when I tape my speech it is difficult to keep it under control for long.

Some stutterers have no difficulty at all speaking when alone, and some have more difficulty than I do. The fact that people stutter when freed from audience pressures is hard to explain, but it may be that some are so conditioned to connect speaking with anxiety that the stress builds up, feeds back to the speech, and disrupts co-ordination.

Some stutterers are said to have controlled their stuttering by standing on mountain tops or lonely beaches and declaiming loudly and at length to imaginary audiences. One winter I tried this on Ben Macdhui, a mountain in Scotland, and startled a flock of white ptarmigan, which crackled away to cries of, 'Go-back, go-back, go-back.' I followed their suggestion, but my speech was no better.

Why do you stutter in some situations and not in others?

Whenever a stutterer approaches a speech situation and begins to speak he must deal with the anxieties and uncertainties that affect his speech. Memories of penalties, frustrations, situation fears, and difficult words or sounds initiate and increase these anxieties. For decades I was as conditioned as Pavlov's dog to go into a major block whenever a taxi driver requested my destination or a telephone operator asked for my name and number. I was reacting to old memories of repeated speech failures in these situations. Some people with speech handicaps, battered by parental, teacher, and peer disapproval, develop feelings of guilt and low self-regard ('What a fool I am not to be able to speak!'). Others, shunned by society and bolted in their glass towers, become filled with frustration, anger, and hostility. All these emotions affect the speech.

The importance of the spoken message can affect a person's fluency. Many stutterers when faced by a life-or-death situation that can only be resolved verbally, are rendered mute. Others, like myself, become completely fluent. Most find that the more important the words, the worse the speech.

Fortunately, there are factors that improve the speech. A

stutterer with high self-regard, good morale, and confidence in himself can bulldoze his way through difficult speaking situations. Success breeds success, and the more fluent a stutterer feels, the more fluent he tends to become.

Charles Van Riper[11] of Western Michigan University combined these factors into a simple model:

$$S = \frac{PFAGH + SfWf + Cs}{M + Fl}$$

where S is the frequency and severity of stuttering, P is penalties; F, frustrations; A, anxiety; G, guilt; H, hostility; Sf, situation fears caused by old memories; Wf, word fear; Cs, communication content; M, morale or confidence; and Fl, amount of felt fluency.

This looks complicated, but all it means is that the factors on the top line increase the stutter and those below the line reduce the stutter. An individual may not feel that all of these factors apply to him, but most will admit that P, F, Sf, and Wf play a major part in their speech control. My main problems were always Sf and Cs, but I managed to develop a strong M which enabled me to communicate fairly well.

Different speaking situations bring different factors to bear on the speech, and a stutterer cannot always predict which emotions will develop and how powerful they will be. Sometimes he starts to speak sure that he is going to block and yet is remarkably fluent. At other times he feels confident and becomes speechless. Good therapy helps him to control his speech even when he is buffeted by conflicting influences and feelings; but without therapy his speech is vulnerable to even minor changes in circumstances or attitude. The answer to the question about why people stutter in some situations and not in others is locked in the labyrinths of our brains.

Will you always stutter? Won't it just go away?

In my case I can be fairly sure that my stutter will not just go away. Although I may learn to control it to the point of 90 per cent fluency, I shall always stutter. This does not apply to everybody. In many cases, particularly in young people, a stutter disappears of its own accord.

Stuttering usually begins in childhood, and between 42 and 81 per cent of children who develop the impediment spontaneously lose it.[12] The age of recovery varies, but some experts feel there is a tendency for stuttering to disappear between the ages of thirteen and twenty years. Studies in Britain suggested a far earlier recovery, and, in one town, a third of the children recovered from transient stuttering by the age of four.[13] The statistics are confused by differences in criteria of what constitutes stuttering. Some so-called early stuttering may have been within the range of normal childish disfluency. Nevertheless, it is safe to say that about half the stutters developed in early childhood more or less disappear, and that spontaneous recovery tends to occur with children who have the less severe speech problems, as you would expect.[14] The reasons for spontaneous recovery are far from clear.

Even stutterers who recover completely, or rapidly improve, can deteriorate in conditions of stress. My own stutter began to fade and caused me few inconveniences between the ages of thirteen and eighteen. However, three years of exposure to the stresses, bangs, and bumps of war caused a steady deterioration in my speech, until I was barely able to communicate at all.

Even in moments of intense anxiety a stutter can have its funny side. A colleague and I were crouching in a slit trench while the opposition noisily tried to turn us into a protein mulch. I kept saying, 'Oh sh____, sh____. Oh sh____, sh____,' until my friend yelled in my ear, 'Telling 'em to shush won't stop them, you idiot!'

'I'm not shushing,' I roared back, angrily and fluently. 'I'm trying to say "Oh shit!" '

Does forcing a left-handed child to use his right hand make him stutter?

My usual reply is that there is no solid evidence that forcing right-handedness on a left-handed child causes a stutter, but my position is undermined a little by the fact that I am ambidextrous, can write with both hands, and got into trouble at school when I held a mug in my left hand!

Early societies tended to look askance at left-handed people as abnormal members of society. The grim word 'sinister' means left. Even in the opening decades of this century there were campaigns in the United States to abolish left-handedness in public schools by compulsion. Early surveys of schools in London, England, revealed that 17 per cent of congenitally left-handed children forced to write with their right hands developed stutters, suggesting that shifting handedness caused the stuttering.[15] Results from later research conflicted with this view; some of the 'shifted' stutterers had developed the impediment before they learned to write.[16]

Since then, a great deal of conflicting information has been collected. The general conclusion reached by Bloodstein in his review of left-handedness and stuttering is that, although some scientists still feel that in some cases a shift of handedness may contribute to the onset of stuttering, stutterers do not differ from non-stutterers in their handedness.[17] Nevertheless, the asymmetry of the brain is still regarded by some scientists as one possible root of the complex problem.

How does a person with a severe stutter cope with life?

My response to this is 'Remarkably well considering the circumstances!' This is not true for people who stutter very severely and have no marketable skills or characteristics that society values. They can be very lonely and unhappy and usually find it hard to get jobs.

In order to survive and do well a person who stutters badly must be determined, skilful, and courageous. He must learn to deal several times a day with traumatic situations that would seriously impair the confidence, self-regard, and even mental health of many people with normal speech. The stutterer strives to maintain his self-esteem and to ignore the adverse responses of other people to his handicap. Some stutterers may appear to be arrogant, but it is usually a reflection of their survival equipment.

Although therapists deplore stutterers' attempts to avoid situations because of their disfluency, it is necessary to be realistic. A severe stutterer would be a fool (and a pauper) if he were to embark on a career as a criminal lawyer. Most of us choose our vocations with care, taking into account our interests, skills, and vocal capabilities; even so, it is not easy and can go awry. One stutterer trained to become an expert on Shakespeare, but found it impossible to get a job in his field and went into horticulture. Another qualified in economics and became a store clerk. The vocal demands of various professions may push stutterers into jobs they did not originally want.

Stutterers tend to plan their day's activities carefully. This is possible if you can allocate your own time and do things at your own pace in your own way, but few of us enjoy those luxuries. I used to go over all the speech situations I was likely to meet and design ways of dealing with them. Many people who stutter have told me how they begin every day with cold, stomach-churning fear of the many foreseeable situations they know they cannot handle. As one man said to me, 'You take your fear of speaking to bed with you, it greets you when you wake in the morning, and it walks beside you all the day.' Stutterers are experts at dealing with fear, anxiety, and rejection.

I was at a scientific conference in Spain where a Dutchman read an excellent scientific paper in English. He had a stutter and was nervous, but coped by using speech techniques effectively. There were a few fifteen-second pauses as he collected his speech and calmed his nerves, but they did not interfere unduly with the flow of information. It was an incredibly good performance. A couple of young Ivy League Americans were sitting beside me, the kind of born-again laboratory scientists who think that only they and their work are of any consequence. They began to laugh, and one of them said, 'The stuttering fool's wasting our time!'

I gave myself ten seconds to curb the flare of anger, then leaned across and burned their ears long and fluently. I pointed out that since neither of them had the professionalism to look beyond the stutter and listen to the useful paper, or the humanity to admire the way the speaker coped with his impediment, they were more handicapped than he was. They walked out of the meeting.

Someone once said, 'Show me a stutterer and I'll show you an angry man.' It is not true to say that stutterers are usually angry people, but they all have to learn to control their tempers when faced by rudeness and brutality. You can't go around modifying people's facial topography all the time.

Small boys who stutter severely are inclined to explode from frustration and punch the nearest tormentor. My father was understandably annoyed when a parent sent him a large dentist's bill for restructuring the front teeth of a son who had had the poor judgment to mimic my stuttering.

People who stutter develop extra keen senses in the same manner that blind people have acutely sensitive touch and hearing. Some stutterers tend to develop the non-verbal components of communication to such an extent that their acute interpretation of body language and synthesis of visual factors can be mistaken for telepathy. A few stuttering individuals can read eye, face, hand, and body signals so well that they have earned their living on the stage as so-called mind readers. This acute visual awareness makes some stutterers foresee people's needs and sense what is going to happen before it happens to an extent that can be disturbing.

Not many stutterers use their impediment deliberately to avoid situations. I did so once, to avoid being forced by the bilingual program in Canada to spend a year away from my research learning French, which I would seldom use. I knew a young soldier who in sheer desperation deliberately increased his stutter and tics to a grotesque degree to discourage a predatory woman with wedding bells ringing in her ears.

Fortunately people can carry on and live under unbelievable hardships. Some stutterers bend beneath the weight of their struggles to speak, while others look upon their stuttering as a challenge and become stronger than most people with normal speech. Nietzsche once wrote, 'That which does not kill me, makes me stronger.' Provided life, or even a handicap, has meaning, people can cope despite pain and deprivation.

Has the stutter held you back in life?

All the severe stutterers who discussed with me the extent to which their impediment controls their lives were unanimous in the view that stuttering hindered their progress more than anything else. I agreed with them until I was asked by my therapist to make a presentation to about forty people about how my stuttering had affected my life.

Before the presentation I drew up a flow-chart, like a good scientist, and examined the main factors that had determined my career decisions and my life's directions. To my great surprise I found that, although the stuttering had caused me many frustrations and problems, it had affected the direction of my life much less than a minor defect in my vision and my inherited personality. The defective eyesight prevented me from going to a naval academy at fourteen years of age and later barred me from becoming a fighter pilot. It probably saved my life. My personality is optimistic, and I more or less ignored my impediment when making career decisions. If people let me – which sometimes they don't – I just cope with the problems my stuttering causes as they crop up.

Although I more or less flunked my public-speaking test by getting the jitters, the presentation helped me to see my handicap objectively. This, I suspect, was the real intention of my crafty therapist.

Of course a stutter is important in a person's career, but it is only one of many influences. Personal skills and character can still be the main influences on lifestyle even when a person cannot communicate effectively.

Does a stutter affect your health?

I chaired a meeting on one of those days when my speech was in an unpredictable downswing. Afterwards a friend asked, 'Does a stutter hurt?' and I replied, 'No, of course not, although the tension can give me a headache.' This was followed by another question asking whether or not stuttering affects a person's health. I replied, 'Probably,' without any solid evidence to support me.

You don't have to be a physician to know that exposure to excessive stress for long periods can undermine your health. Stress is all very well in its place and can be the spice of life, but when it occurs too often and too strongly and is accompanied by frustration and anxiety, the spice tends to turn sour. The stresses caused by stuttering are not always of the healthy kind.

Early research on stuttering focused on physiological and psychological phenomena, but few reports discuss the possible effects on general health and longevity. During stuttering there can be antagonism between abdominal and thoracic breathing and irregularity of breathing cycles. When a stutterer blocks, breathing can cease.[18] I once saw a stutterer faint from a prolonged block; he just ran out of oxygen. During stuttering there is often an acceleration of the heart rate and a change in the distribution of the blood, as well as a decrease in the blood's total sugar and blood protein.[19] Surprisingly, little definitive information about the blood pressure of stutterers was located, although many of the middle-aged male stutterers I meet suffer to some extent from hypertension – which is to be expected in a frequently stressed person.

These symptoms arise in non-stutterers when they are excited or stressed, but people who stutter are exposed to excessive stress so often that it seems likely that their health will be affected in the long run. It would be interesting to see figures comparing the incidence of hypertension and heart complaint in middle-aged stutterers and non-stutterers. You are probably better off without a stutter as far as your general health is concerned.

Does it help to speak slowly?

Yes, it does. Most stutterers try to speak far too quickly as they try to get the words over with before they stumble and block. For a stutterer, speaking quickly is about as wise as running over ground strewn with jagged boulders in the dark instead of picking his way carefully step by step. He's likely to fall painfully on his fanny.

Most people speak at a rate of about 150 to 200 words per minute (wpm), although two of my daughters communicate in a verbal deluge of 200 to 300 wpm. Most untreated stutterers try to get out about 150 wpm or more when most of them can only cope with 60 wpm or less. The majority of speech pathologists start treatment by reducing the patient's speech rate to 30 to 40 wpm, and most stutterers can keep fluent in the clinic at these rates if they prolong their words. Unfortunately, prolonged speech at 30 wpm is a little bizarre and not really socially acceptable; although, as the therapists say, it's far better than going into a block, running out of breath, twitching, and closing your eyes as you fight to ask the way to the washroom.

Reducing speech rate is not as easy as it sounds. All people delude themselves about how fast they talk. I sat for days with a stop-watch and tape recorder before I managed to bring my speech rate down from a torrential 200 wpm to 60 wpm or less. The slow speech sounded like a 78 rpm record played at 33 rpm, but I was much more fluent. After a while I learned to feel my speech rate. When I felt tension entering my speech, I knew that I was exceeding my optimum speech rate of 80 wpm. The speech-rate control worked in the therapy sessions, but it was not the whole answer. Outside the clinic the slow speech was penalized by the startled expressions on listeners' faces and was not rewarded by the beams of approval the heavy-footed words earned in the clinic.

One bit of advice will help both stutterers and clutterers. Speak slowly and smoothly, on oiled wheels, as slowly as you can. It won't harm and it could be a great help.

Technology has entered the picture with an electronic speech-rate monitor called the Hector Speech Aid.[20] The principle is that when a person who stutters speaks too quickly, the gadget emits a warning tone. The aim is to help those who have difficulty feeling their speech rate to regulate their speech speed, and to remind people like myself to slow down when they begin to gabble. I am considering buying each of my fast-talking daughters one of these speech-rate monitors for Christmas.

Can a stutter be cured?

The simple answer is that it is unlikely that an adult with a severe, long-established stutter will ever be *completely* cured by the clinical methods available today. Young children and adolescents may be 'cured,' but not adults.

This is not as gloomy as it sounds, because most people who stutter can, if they co-operate fully, be taught to control their stuttering to the extent that it is no longer a social embarrassment or a handicap in the workplace. They can learn to communicate without major interruptions and express their thoughts and feelings much more freely. Every year scientists gain deeper insights into stuttering and more patients respond to better treatment. The sooner a person with a stutter comes for treatment, the more the clinicians can help him. The various treatments for stuttering are described in a later chapter. Here it suffices to say that a person with a very severe stutter (like mine) can be helped more than he imagines in his wildest dreams. The future is bright.

People will come up with other, more difficult questions. It is hoped that the rest of this book will provide a few of the answers.

THREE

The bending of the twig

' 'Tis education forms the common mind.
Just as the twig is bent, the tree's inclined.'

Alexander Pope

The roots of most stuttering reach down into early childhood. The problem can begin when the child utters his first stumbling words and solicitous parents lean over the crib and marvel at the cleverness of such a morsel of humanity in being able to speak so clearly. They may encourage or even pressure the babe to say more words as clearly as possible as soon as possible and lovingly marvel at his precocity, thereby sowing the seeds of a stutter. These seeds may or may not germinate and grow. It depends upon the child.

People are prone to jump to the conclusion that all stutters were caused by unhappy childhoods. Many stutterers can remember being unhappy when they were children, but so can many people who don't have problems with their speech. In any case, happiness is hard to define, and expecting early childhood to be free from stress and frustration is unrealistic.

There are volumes of learned papers about the frequency of stuttering in people of different ages, social levels, and races. The findings of the scientists are contradictory, but there is a common thread running through the reports. There is good evidence that stuttering is frequent in societies that expect children to conform to rigid patterns of behaviour and to develop and display speaking skills when very young. Stutters seem to flourish where social pressures are brought to bear early in life, and it is fair to say that stuttering is to some extent a social complaint.

Pressures on young children

If young children were to be freed from all social pressures and strictures there would be anarchy in the nursery. Little twigs need to be gently bent to grow in directions that will make them happy, useful, and acceptable members of society. The question is how to do so without creating fertile ground in which stuttering and other problems can develop.

Those of us who were raised in the first third of this century were encouraged to read worthy books designed to hammer into our heads the Victorian ideals of courage, honour, truth, duty, and other virtues now regarded as outmoded, while our teachers gave us ample opportunity to develop and demonstrate stoicism as they whacked the same values into our other ends. One of the best pictures of those days is found in Desmond Coke's *The Bending of the Twig*, a book that describes dispassionately how boys were painfully but effectively moulded into the form demanded by a strict society. It was the way things were. Few people, not even the children, regarded the process as unkind.

Books of this genre show that it was perfectly normal to force children to conform to clearly defined patterns of behaviour, and pressures like these persist to this day in different and less physical forms. Modern educators condemn the corporal disciplining of children in the earlier school systems as brutal and uncivilized, but some modern, so-called psychological methods of disciplining a child through peer pressure, ridicule, and guilt can be no less brutal. The application of intense emotional pressure can inflict lasting pain. In the old system, the person who was most feared and hated was not the teacher with the switch but the one with a sarcastic, cutting tongue who could shrivel a child's self-respect to the size of a peanut with a few carefully chosen words. Pressures are pressures whether they are physical or mental.

Competitive Western society has never been particularly kind to its children, and intense pressures to behave in certain ways are still brought to bear as soon as the umbilical cord has been cut. There are people who expose the developing foetus to high levels of oxygen in the hope that the child will become a genius. Pressures on a young child begin at home, but they immediately escalate when apprehensive small fry are thrown into the educational fish pond where they are urged to communicate well in public and to *Achieve* with a capital 'A.'

Contrary to what most school children think, teachers are ordinary people trying to do a job as best they can. Some are kind, some are indifferent, and a few are brutally sadistic. The majority mean well. It is curious, therefore, that a number of stuttering adults I have met felt that, although other children could be cruel, the ridicule and insensitivity of their teachers caused their worst problems. Even today I hear hair-raising stories about teachers' thoughtless cruelty to children slightly handicapped by impaired speech, or sight, or hearing but not enough to warrant special education. The cruelty most frequently takes the shape of ridicule. The stuttering child may be made the class scapegoat, or may thoughtlessly be asked to carry out tasks that, because of his partial handicap, are beyond his capabilities. 'Partial' is the key word; teachers can deal with someone who is completely mute, deaf, or blind. They simply send him to a specialist.

Most teachers who maltreat handicapped children are not vicious, cruel people. They merely suffer from insensitivity, impatience, and a shortage of time to think about and allow for a child's physical and mental shortcomings. I clearly remember being taken to task at the age of eight when I biffed an impatient, frustrated English teacher on her belly-button for mimicking my speech. She sat down on the floor and displayed to all the class her thick, dark-blue knickers, which were secured by yellow ribbons just above her knees. She was, in fact, a nice person, but she never forgave me.

If you have a stutter, a funny accent, a long nose, sticky-out teeth, big ears, a wandering eye, slightly webbed feet, a slight limp, or a facial lump, or are fat, skinny, or unusual in any way and have not been unduly penalized in the safe co-coon of home, you soon will be when you go to school. Young children are likely to chomp their milk teeth into any companion who has the misfortune to look strange or act differently from the herd. Sending a stuttering child to school is like throwing a kitten into the dog pound, but the kitten must take its chances in the mêlée of life and develop sufficient agility and sharp enough claws to survive.

School is tough even for children who speak normally. Those who stutter are under greater pressure than others in the school system, and this tends to make the stuttering worse. Today, teachers are more understanding and better trained than when I was at school, and there are often speech therapists (albeit overworked ones) to assist the school's staff. Nevertheless, the child must still cope with the classroom jungle. Some stuttering children accept defeat and leave school early. Those who remain must struggle to survive.

A therapist once asked me what I felt about my early days at school. I replied that it was one long fight. Most stutterers I have met feel the same.[1]

Stuttering in primitive societies

Some primitive societies provide a clue to the relationship between social pressures and the development of stuttering in young children. In some tribes stuttering is rare. There may not even be a word for the disorder in their languages. Investigations of 6,000 people in eight tribes in New Guinea revealed no stutterers, and the impediment appeared to be rare in Australian aborigines. Anthropologist Margaret Mead never saw stuttering in the people of New Guinea and the South Pacific, and in the first half of this century stuttering was unknown in certain groups of Eskimos.[2]

Studies of speech defects of North American Indians provided insights into the effects of social pressures on children. During the 1930s, the Bannock and Shoshone Indians lived on isolated reservations in southeastern Idaho where the impact of European social customs was minimal. John C. Snidecor, who studied these tribes from 1937 to 1939, once asked the tribal council if they knew any stuttering Indians. They didn't have a word for stuttering in their language and didn't know what the researcher was talking about. Snidecor had to demonstrate what stuttering looked and sounded like, and the chiefs thought his antics very funny indeed. Nevertheless, the scientist offered a reward to anybody who could find a *bona fide* stuttering Indian. The hunt was on.[3]

I like to imagine what happened when Snidecor interviewed 800 people and demonstrated stuttering by blocking and repeating to audiences who hadn't the faintest idea what it was all about. There must have been a few hilarious moments. Snidecor had great difficulty finding any Indians with definite stutters.

In these non-stuttering Indian societies there was little or no cultural pressure on children. They were not expected to speak and perform until adolescence and were permitted a great deal of freedom. They were not forced to conform with rigid cultural standards, and a child was not likely to be criticized for the way he spoke. The tribes looked upon speech development as a normal part of growing up, and interference in the process by solicitous parents for purposes of display was not encouraged.[4]

The Indians of the Northwest coast – for example, the Kwakiutl, the Nootka, and the Salish tribes – were just the opposite. Edwin Lemert, a social anthropologist from the University of California, observed large numbers of individuals with stutters in these tribes, which also had words for stuttering in their language and even rituals to treat the disability.[5] Speech defects of this kind were commonplace, and memories of stuttering ancestors went back to the first half of the nineteenth century, before European cultures had much impact.

These tribes, which lived by salmon fishing, were fiercely competitive communities and brought severe pressures to bear on very young children. There were bitter clan rivalries, and so the prestige and status of the clan and its families were of prime importance. People were valued when their prowess reflected favourably on the tribe, and weakness and nonconformity were frowned upon. Young children were expected to comply with clearly defined codes of behaviour and were rigorously taught to participate in public rituals under the critical eye of clan members. Poor verbal delivery, mistakes in procedure, and differences in appearance and behaviour were not acceptable.

People with such handicaps as left-handedness, obesity, smallness, lameness, and impaired speech were treated with scorn and rejected by the clan because they reflected badly on the group. Anybody with hesitant speech must have had a bad time in this competitive, intolerant society. Unfortunately, there are many parallels in modern Western society where competitive tribes tend to develop in the workplace.

Surveys of the stuttering Cowichan Indians of Vancouver Island in Canada and of the non-stuttering Ute Indians supported Lemert's results.[6] The Cowichans, with their stutterers, were competitive and less permissive in child raising than the fluent Utes, who allowed children to develop at their own rates. Stuttering was common in the Idoma and Ibo peoples of West Africa. As many as 2.6 per cent of the Ibos stuttered in a society where verbal communication and the ability to speak in public were important. Orators were greatly admired, and children who were not fluent were slapped and ridiculed by their parents. The people of this highly competitive tribe expected children to be successful in school and provided an environment where a child was likely to develop anxieties about his speech if he were at all disfluent.[7]

Stuttering is known in the Bantu tribe of South Africa and was present before the arrival of white settlers. Bantu and European societies have similar attitudes toward developing fluency, and it is interesting that the frequencies of stuttering (about 1 per cent) in the two societies are similar.[8]

Modern speech pathologists question that there are societies with no stutterers, but there is no doubt that stuttering is much more common in some groups than in others. It is often said that stuttering is more common in Japan than elsewhere, but there is little evidence to support this view. The idea may have originated in a misinterpretation of Lemert's averral that stuttering in Japan is relatively frequent compared with other Pacific societies, where it is rare.

The frequency of stuttering in Japan is an enigma, and estimates vary considerably. Although Japanese children are raised strictly in a conformist society, it has been estimated that about 0.82 per cent of the children stutter.[9] Surprisingly, this is a little less than the average 1 per cent. The Tokyo

Speech Clinic indicated that the data available suggest that only 0.05 per cent of the populace stutter, but felt that the reason for this very low estimate is that Japanese stutterers are ashamed of their hesitancy, tend to hide their problem, don't seek help, and hence are not recorded in the surveys.[10]

Surveys of children show considerable variation from nation to nation and even between towns in the same country. On average about 1 per cent stutter, but in Prague, Czechoslovakia, for example, only 0.55 per cent of 26,000 children stuttered, while 1.82 per cent of 875,384 children studied in Poland stuttered. About 0.93 per cent of the children of a Moslem nation such as Egypt stutter, which is about the same for the Christian society of Denmark (0.90 per cent). The American town of Tuscaloosa, Alabama, had a great many stuttering children (2.12 per cent) in 1973 compared to the Rocky Mountain region (0.30 per cent) in 1969. The stuttering male:female ratio is low in Tuscaloosa (2.7:1) and very high in the Rockies (6:1).[11]

What causes these differences and similarities? Is it the attitude of parents toward their children, the pressures of society, the phonetic complexity of language, or inherited abnormalities? Nobody knows. The answer probably lies in the interaction of many human and environmental factors. Perhaps some day a systems analyst will put it all together in a computer and provide the answer, or at least help us to ask the right questions.

A child is capable of bringing upon himself intense pressures to communicate that could affect his speech before he goes to school, quite apart from pressures from the family and society. I suspect that I was one of these self-starters, because, although my memory goes back to the age of two years, I have no memories of family demands to conform and perform. There was certainly sibling rivalry, and my father was a formidable figure whom we treated with huge respect and addressed with polite caution, but there were few strictures on how we spoke and no penalties for imperfect syntax. Nevertheless, I certainly stuttered when I went to school at the age of five. I couldn't answer my name at roll call on the first day and was soundly spanked for dumb insolence.

I know from my memories and checking with my family

that I was a mentally active child, spilling over with curiosity and wonder about my new world and constantly saying 'Why?' I don't remember anxiety about speaking, but I can still recall the intense frustration of not being able to put my childish thoughts, feelings, and questions into words because I had not yet mastered language and had such a limited vocabulary.

When a child learns that his parents and siblings don't understand what he says, this leads to fears about isolation from the family group. It takes a child time to learn to cope with frustration and isolation. Impeded communication can be as great a pressure as fear of speaking.

Western society, with its increasing emphasis on early achievement and with the high value it places on the spoken word, is a fertile breeding ground for stuttering. Impatience and intolerance are commonplace in the home and workplace. As people strive for material things they tend to ignore human values. An awareness by teachers and parents that early social pressures can damage a child who is only slightly impaired or a little slow to develop would be a start. Unfortunately, many parents and teachers were raised in the pressure-cooker of the Western educational system and, as they survived, cannot see much wrong with it. As the prophet Ezekiel said, when fathers eat sour grapes, the children's teeth are set on edge.

I know a tall husky man with a severe stutter who lives on the rolling farmlands of Ontario. He smiles a great deal and loves to meet people. His outgoing manner helps him to make friends easily. He plays the fiddle, revels in a party, and has great fun with singing roles in amateur theatricals. He enjoys life. As a child he walked a mile or two to school. For several years the bigger boys used to lie in wait for him and beat him up nearly every day, just because he stuttered. At school the busy teacher, impatient with the boy's slowness in answering questions and reading aloud, publicly labelled him stupid. How he managed to grow up into a warm and friendly adult is a mystery.

FOUR

What causes a stutter?

'To harmonize the pressures exerted by society and by the individuals' drives is the greatest problem of human life.'

Abraham Meyerson

Charles Van Riper described the origins of a stutter in terms of a river and its sources.[1] The river is there for all to see, but any attempt to trace it back to its source is complicated by the fact that high up in the hills it is fed by many small streams. It is impossible to say which one is the main source.

A child starts off with his inherited physical and mental equipment – his constitution – which, as the child grows older will be affected by what he experiences and learns. The tempo of life increases, and so does speech development. In these early stages any stuttering problems can be easily treated, but some children get swept along on emotional currents they find hard to control. Gradually, if the speech remains impeded, the child meets frustration and fear and by then is in real trouble. Without help he will be swept by life into the whirlpool of self-reinforcement, where stuttering breeds anxiety, which increases stuttering – a closed cycle that is the unenviable fate of many adults. They can only be rescued by well-designed therapy and great determination.

Although scientists have sought the single cause of a stutter for centuries, most modern experts accept that many factors are involved. Some psychologists still cling to the idea of a single neurotic origin; however, even if such neuroses exist, their effects are likely to be shaped by the pressures of life.

Most people have childhood problems of one kind or another, but most people don't stutter.

Numerous attempts have been made by scientists to find an organic cause for stuttering in, for example, abnormalities of brain structure and/or biochemistry, but the results of research are conflicting. Other authorities favour such so-called non-organic reasons as neuroses, fears of speaking, and faulty speech techniques.

Non-organic phenomena, like neuroses and fear, originate in our brain's chemistry, so that differentiating between organic and non-organic causes of stuttering is fundamentally questionable. Nevertheless, the two categories are useful in that they neatly separate the two therapeutic approaches: the one focusing on a person's physical make-up and the other on his attitudes and speech techniques. The second approach is the most common.

Whether a child is predisposed to stutter by a physical quirk of brain structure and chemistry, which may or may not be triggered by his life's experiences, is still a point in question. Many researchers speak of the 'syndrome' of stuttering, implying a set of symptoms; and this is perhaps the best way to think of a stutter – as a speech abnormality consisting of a set of interacting factors that vary from one person to another. Any attempt to attribute individual causes would be premature, although most speech pathologists have their own private and, so far, unprovable hunches.

There are so many factors that could contribute to the onset of a stutter and perpetuate the impediment that novice speech-therapy students tend to raise their hands in horror and take up some other profession. It is necessary, however, to be aware of these factors in order to understand their complexity and how difficult it is to treat the stutter as a whole.

If at times my tone is irreverent, I offer the plea that some of the theories tested on me did not fit my stutter when I participated as a guinea pig in speech research. Some of the ideas seemed very funny at the time. Nevertheless these theories may fit other stutters much better than mine. While I smile at these ideas, I do not mean to deride them.

According to H.R. Beech and Fay Fransella of the University of London, England, 'Stuttering theory, in general, does not reflect the kind of progressive change and refinement which one might expect from a developing science. To some extent the field may suffer as a result of being treated as one of the social sciences, and perhaps it is the case that the "hard facts" which are necessary to the foundation of a satisfactory science are lacking and difficult to discover.'[2] A friend who is a frustrated speech pathologist stated this much more succinctly: 'It's a can of worms!'

The labyrinth of the mind

Psychologists have theorized for nearly a century about the possibility that stuttering is an expression of urgent but unconscious needs with roots in the nursing and toilet-training stages of development and in the earliest and most primitive of a baby's satisfactions. The 'Repressed Need Theory' is that a stutterer unconsciously wishes to stutter in order to gratify these unconscious needs. This is probably the origin of the incautious layman's belief that a stutterer can choose not to stutter. He inflicts his stutter on himself because he wants to – so let him get on with it! Even if the repressed need theory were correct, the wish would be unconscious, and a stutterer would need lengthy psychotherapy to consciously control it. This theory *may* apply to *some* stutterers, since people stutter for such a variety of reasons, including psychological abnormality, abnormal brain structure and function, and physical injury.

Psychoanalysis of many stutterers has produced no conclusive evidence one way or the other that stuttering originates from a repression of infantile needs. For a while this theory was very much in vogue. It was the basis of treatment of stuttering and many other disabilities, but is less widely accepted today. We are all products of our genes, chemistry, experience, and environment. Events, emotions, and needs encountered during our early childhood affect us for the rest of our lives. Whether we like it or not, the small child exists within us even though we may not recognize it as such. We learn to live with it. As Nietzsche wrote, 'In every real man a child is hidden that wants to play.'

Memories of infantile needs may affect a stutter – since

practically every emotion and change in environment seem to do so – but labelling repressed need as the main or sole cause of stuttering seems to be unjustified. It may be one of the numerous tributaries feeding the mainstream of the stutter, but it is not likely to be the main source of the whole river.

Shortly after World War II a grateful government offered to pay psychoanalysts to seek out the cause of my severe stutter if I would act as a guinea pig for the mind-benders. An official made it quite clear that it would be good for me, like a dose of Epsom Salts. He left no doubt in my mind that he thought that anyone who stuttered was nuts. Since I was between jobs, as it were, and the expense allowance was attractive, I accepted.

My mentor was a serious, unsmiling young man, full to overflowing with the teachings of good old Sigmund Freud. It was a period when psychologists and psychiatrists tended to see everything you said, dreamed, or did in terms of Freudian symbolism. After the long period of Victorian taboos about mentioning any part of the anatomy lower than the chin, Freud gave people a marvellous reason to talk about their reproductive bits and pieces. Freud doubtless brought mental health out of the Dark Ages, but he would be horrified if he could see how many of his disciples have gone overboard in their interpretation of his theories when there is so little evidence to support their views.

North America adopted these ideas with such enthusiasm that every flag-pole, cigar, or linear object came under suspicion as a symbol of some dark and sexy motivation. Maybe that's why church steeples went out of fashion in most of Canada and the United States and were replaced by horrible, soulless triangles and cubes of no possible naughty significance. (The exception is, of course, Quebec. French Canadians kept their steeples, which will doubtless give Freudian sociologists something to write doctoral theses about.)

When I started the analysis I soon learned that the difference between a psychologist and a psychiatrist is that the latter can stick needles in you and the former can't. Within a short time I became a pincushion.

At one session my serious young man pumped me full of pentothal. As I floated on a warm, comfortable, carefree

cloud, he asked me a strange question. I read the transcript
later and I remember my replies clearly:

DOCTOR: Now just relax. *(I was already paralysed.)* Can you
hear me?

ME: Mmmm.

DOCTOR: Tell me, now, which of your testicles is lower than
the other?

ME: You're joking?

DOCTOR: No, this is serious. Please tell me.

ME: *(Silence)*

DOCTOR: What's wrong?

ME: I'm thinking. Wouldn't you?

DOCTOR: Come along now. Surely you know.

ME: I haven't the faintest idea.

DOCTOR: Nonsense! You must know. We *all* know.

ME: Do you know which of yours is lowest?

DOCTOR: That's beside the point.

ME: I couldn't put it better myself. *(Low chuckle)*

DOCTOR: *(Long silence)* Try to remember. Haven't you ever
looked?

ME: I just don't know. I guess I've never looked that
closely.

DOCTOR: You've never looked? Oh come now! Can you tell
me if you have two of them?

ME: My God! Are you implying I've got more than
two? I *demand* a recount!

End of session. In fact, it was the end of the experiment because he said that I was the only patient he knew who could
crack jokes, argue, and tell downright lies when I was nearly
unconscious. I was not a suitable guinea pig.

The real reason for my ignorance about my anatomy was
that in the Armed Forces the only mirror I possessed was very
small, bent, and made of scratched polished steel. I used it
for shaving. It was not designed for wider surveys.

My young analyst was hot on the track of things like repressed needs and low self-awareness, but I was a grave disappointment to him because he found remarkably little
wrong with my mental health. I learned a great deal about

myself and the way the human mind works, and both have been invaluable. I shall always be grateful to him even when I chuckle at his expense.

Supporters of the repressed need theory have several arrows in their quiver. They feel that a stutter may satisfy an infantile need to recall the oral gratifications of breast-feeding; may attempt to satisfy anal erotic needs by recalling infantile satisfactions; or may hide hostile feelings that the person who stutters is scared to display. They hypothesize that the stutterer chews words in order symbolically to cannibalize his parents; or achieves silence in the face of social pressures to speak in order to avoid uttering obscenities.[3] However, many stutterers I know have no trouble at all uttering four-letter words when they are angry. Adults with anal obsessions apparently exhibit excessive moral rectitude, punctuality, stinginess, and orderliness, whereas most of the stutterers I know are messy, generous, not excessively moral, and not particularly punctual. The hat doesn't seem to fit. These anal characteristics are, however, a fair definition of what is generally required in a good public servant.

The scientific evidence suggests that the average stutterer is not unusually neurotic or severely maladjusted. He doesn't appear to have any special characteristics that set him apart from non-stutterers except his strange way of speaking. Some stutterers may not be so well adjusted to society as non-stutterers; and some do suffer from low self-esteem, anxiety, hostility, and an unwillingness to take risks. All these are to be expected considering the nature of the impediment and the frequently adverse responses of society to disfluency.

It is important to bear in mind that while no fundamental neurosis has been shown to be a general cause of stuttering, all people who stutter severely experience fear of speaking, anxiety, and frustration every day of their lives. These powerful emotions are integral parts of stuttering, and their control is of vital importance in therapy. It is here that the psychiatrists and psychologists have an important role to play.

In the previous chapter the relationship between stuttering and societies where children are expected to speak, perform, conform, and achieve at a very early age was discussed. There seems little doubt that social pressures and the fears arising from them are involved in the development of stuttering. This is, however, a matter of conscious fear and is not to be confused with such deeply rooted Freudian neuroses as unconscious repressed needs.

All of us are beset by mental problems every day. The important thing is how our problems manifest themselves and how we deal with them. Many seemingly normal people are handicapped by tremendous secret inner conflicts. The trouble with stuttering is that it is there for all to see whenever you speak.

Is stuttering inherited?

Stuttering parents often have stuttering offspring, but there is little concrete evidence that stuttering is inherited. Nevertheless, according to some scientists, recent evidence suggests that biological inheritance may play some role in stuttering. I know several stuttering parents with stuttering sons, but I also know many more stutterers, including myself, who have no other people with stutters in their family trees. Many non-stutterers have stuttering children. It is all too easy to jump to unsupported conclusions.

Parental attitudes and their effect on the way a child feels about speech may account for stuttering that runs in families. A parent who stutters is sure to be anxious about speaking. It goes with the territory. A stuttering parent is also likely to be apprehensive about a child's normal, early, stumbling speech as he learns to talk. There is always the fear that the child's minor disfluencies will develop into the stuttering that caused the parent so much anxiety and frustration. Unless the parent is sufficiently well-informed to be able to tell the difference between normal, childish disfluency and the tension, avoidance, and fear of words of a true stutter, he may try to correct the child, and punish him whenever he struggles to form words and sentences. There are many heartbreaking stories about stuttering parents slapping their children every time their speech stumbled in desperate attempts to spare the children their lifelong pain. Early association of fear, pain, disapproval, and anxiety with speaking is likely to increase a child's risk of becoming disfluent.

From 23 to 69 per cent of people who stutter have family histories of stuttering, while 1.3 to 42 per cent of non-stutterers have family histories of stuttering.[4] The two sets of percentages overlap considerably.

A detailed study was made of a family in Iowa in which 40 per cent of the family members stuttered. The family tree showed five generations of stutterers. The members were exceedingly conscious of their speech and believed their disorder was inherited. A genetic and social analysis indicated that the stuttering in the Iowa family arose from the fact that the family members themselves falsely diagnosed normal, early speech disfluencies as stuttering and acted accordingly. Twenty years after the stuttering family had been counselled about the problem only one in forty-four of the family stuttered.[5]

The fact that children develop stutters when raised away from their parents in communal institutions, such as *kibbutzim* in Israel, where they receive objective upbringing, has been interpreted as refuting the theory of environmental (i.e., parental) triggering of stuttering. Nevertheless, objective schooling away from the parents usually involves persuading the child to conform with institutional rather than parental standards in early life; the pressures may be different, but they are still there. Life in an institution is not usually warm-hearted and supportive. Even the word 'objective' has a cold ring to it.

If a predisposition to stuttering is inherited, it is likely to be controlled by many genes (polygenic inheritance) rather than by only one. Genes can interact with each other and with the environment. The factors that produce a stutter are exceedingly complex.

The occurrence of disorders in twins is a useful tool for probing whether a malady is controlled by the genes in our chromosomes. The classic case is schizophrenia. It has been known for many years that the average person has about a 1 per cent chance of developing schizophrenia, while the identical twin of a schizophrenic has a 50 per cent chance of developing the complaint. If a child is schizophrenic and has a non-identical twin, this twin has a 15 per cent chance of being schizophrenic. The same applies to non-twin brothers and sisters.[6]

Many studies of twins have been unsatisfactory because of small samples, inappropriate procedures, and differences in the way parents treat identical and non-identical twins. Seymour Kety and his colleagues in Massachusetts were aware of these shortcomings when they made a careful study of 5,000 adopted 20- to 45-year-old twins in Denmark.[7] Thirty-three of these people were schizophrenic and twenty-eight of the latter had been adopted as babies. The researchers located thirty-three non-schizophrenic adopters with similar backgrounds and surveyed the relatives of both schizophrenic and non-schizophrenic groups. None of the original, biological relatives of non-schizophrenic adopted children had schizophrenia, and the incidences of schizophrenia in the adoptive parents of adopted schizophrenics and non-schizophrenics were similar (2 to 4 per cent). As many as 10 per cent of the biological relatives of the schizophrenic adopters had schizophrenia. This carefully controlled experiment demonstrated that schizophrenia is genetically mediated.

It is well known that up to 13 per cent of individuals in twin pairs have stutters compared with about 1 per cent of the normal population. Conversely, 4.5 per cent of 461 stutterers studied had a twin, compared with 1.2 per cent in 500 non-stutterers. There is good reason to assume that stuttering and twinning are linked.

Although some researchers feel that this link between twinning and stuttering is genetic,[8] not all researchers are convinced that there is solid proof that stuttering is an inherited disorder. Stuttering develops in response to childhood pressures and stresses, whatever the initial cause. If one twin (particularly a close, identical twin) stutters severely, the other is likely to associate anxiety with speech and to be more likely to stutter than others. Identical twins are treated alike, and any censure of a stuttering member of the pair is likely to be felt by the other.

When a child is adopted and still develops a stutter, if he has a family history of stuttering it is easy to jump to the conclusion that, since he has been raised away from the influence of his stuttering parents or siblings, he is genetically predisposed to stutter and is responding to genes rather than to environment. Unfortunately, human nature again muddies the water. Not all people want to adopt a stuttering child or a child with a family history of stuttering. There is a tendency for people who stutter or who have stuttering relatives to be more sympathetic to a disfluent child and more ready to take him under their wing. Since such adoptive parents are aware of budding stuttering symptoms, they are also likely to check the child's speech, so that he may well develop a stutter in his new, sympathetic surroundings.

Bloodstein studied twelve adopted stutterers, and in only three cases was there stuttering in the adoptive family.[9] Again, this small sample suggests a possible hereditary basis, but genetic analysis of large stuttering families does not support this view. Conclusive evidence could be obtained from a rigorous, large-scale investigation of adopted, stuttering twins and their families similar to that carried out by Kety and his colleagues to confirm the genetic basis of schizophrenia. Perhaps the information already exists in Kety's files and just awaits analysis. His team studied 5,000 individuals and 4,967 of these were non-schizophrenic. In general about 1 per cent of people in Europe stutter, so about 50 of Kety's sample, including twins, would stutter. A survey of the incidence of stuttering in the biological and adoptive families of the stuttering twins and a comparable sample of non-stuttering twins would settle once and for all whether stuttering, or the predisposition to it, is mediated by genes.

The tools used to study whether stuttering is a genetic disorder have been relatively crude, and most of the discussions focus on how much of the stutter is genetically and how much environmentally caused. Even if stuttering is a genetic disorder, it is likely to be affected by the environment one way or the other. The gene effects could be very subtle, because chemicals (e.g., a steroid latched onto another molecule within our body) can effect the patterns by which ribonucleic acid (RNA, involved in our energy supply) and protein (e.g., enzyme) are produced without interfering with heredity. The influences of the genes are therefore liable to be blown on different courses by the winds of chemical mediation.[10]

When you consider how complex is the development of the nerve patterns in our brains during the growth of the human foetus, and how even minor defects – in the chemical gradients, in the attractions and rejections of our immune system, in the microscopic brain structures that guide the developing threadlike axons, and in the chemistry of the neurotransmitters at the synaptic connections – can cause major behavioural defects, it is a miracle that more of us don't suffer from major abnormalities of the nervous system.

Even when the nerve network is established, it can be changed by the environment. People used to think that human behaviour was quite distinct from genetics and that, although we can inherit eye and hair colour, the environment and how we react to it determines what we do. Many biologists now feel that this is incorrect and that minor differences in genes and their effects on the nervous system can strongly determine our behaviour.

Can anxiety be inherited?

There is little doubt that anxiety has a major effect on the fluency of an adult with a severe stutter, and it is fair to ask whether anxiety or fearfulness can be inherited. It appears that it can be – at least in dogs, which don't differ a great deal from people in their chemistry.

John P. Scott and John L. Fuller studied the genetics of behaviour in cocker spaniels and basenjis. Spaniels are bred for their responses to hand signals and for the soft mouths necessary for game retrieval. The dogs have a long history of benevolent association with man. Basenjis are tough hunting dogs that were used by pygmies and other Africans in a much less kindly manner.

Both types of dog were crossed and back-crossed and examined for the amount of aggression they showed in play and for their fearfulness. The evidence strongly indicated that both aggressive play and fearfulness were inherited, the former being controlled by two genes and the latter by one gene. The pure basenji pups were much more playfully aggressive at three to four months than the pure spaniels. While the spaniels were at ease with man, five-week-old basenji pups showed their fear of people by yelping, snapping, and running away. This fear subsided later, but the basenjis were always more restless than the spaniels.[11]

Since youthful anxiety appears to be heritable, how does this apply to a stutter? Anxiety about speaking could be genetically controlled, but if this is the case, why do so many stutters spontaneously disappear? In the case of the basenji pups, they lost most of their inherited fear when they learned to trust people and expect kindness from them. It is possible that stuttering children lose their stutters when the world treats them kindly, while those who feel the full weight of society's censure develop intractable, persistent, self-reinforcing stutters. This is, of course, sheer speculation, but the possibility of inherited speech-related anxiety and the development from it of an anxiety-conditioned speech disability cannot be ignored.

Would we expect speech to be conditioned by anxiety during man's evolution? Yes, we probably would. Ever since early man learned to speak and found that what he said to his peers could, if sufficiently ill-advised, get his hair parted by a Neanderthal club, he would be inclined to get hang-ups about speaking. He would be disposed to watch what he said and lapse into fractured speech the moment someone disapproved – unless, of course, he was the best club wielder in the tribe. Anxiety is closely associated with hesitant communication, even when people have normal speech. There remains the knotty problem of why more men stutter than vocally precocious females. Maybe our ancestors were reluctant to bash their breeding woman and learned to put up with their early verbosity.

All this speculation is on shaky foundations, and some scientists are sceptical about the sociobiologists' claim that behaviour can be inherited. Nevertheless, it is possible that whether a stutter is genetically mediated is not just a matter of abnormal genes directly affecting the stutterer's vocal motor system and musculature. It may be much more subtle – so subtle, in fact, that the elementary techniques used so far could not possibly recognize the defects. If a stutter proves to be genetically controlled, it would be as well for researchers to focus on how the genes affect the stutter at a chemical level, rather than debate how much is genetically and how much environmentally caused.

If we accept that anxiety and behaviour may be inherited, we need to buy a larger can to accommodate all the new, fat, and active worms.

Since a stutter is so complex, why bother to probe it in depth? Schizophrenia is a complex disability; but when it was discovered that it was controlled by genes, and when its processes were understood better, it was possible to help many schizophrenics with neuroleptic drugs to block the receptors of dopamine (a neurotransmitter) in the gaps between the nerve cells (synapses).

Nevertheless, I believe that the debate between the organic and non-organic schools of thought about the origins of stuttering is futile. Whether stuttering is an organic disorder is beside the point. All our anticipatory fears about speech and our avoidances are chemically controlled in the enzymatic stew of our brain's limbic system and its links with our speech and motor centres. How many times does a stuttering child face the choice between 'fight or flight' in a difficult speaking situation and respond blindly from his old brain inherited from reptilian ancestors? Are the sudden fear and response inorganic? They are not.

Although there is still no clear evidence that stuttering is inherited, modern science is leaning toward the idea that genetic factors are involved. Studies are hindered by the difficulty of distinguishing between childish disfluency and an early stutter, by the fact that many attributes of a stutter are hard to measure, and by the complex effects of emotional factors on fluency. If many genes are involved, and the environment can affect their expression, the researchers must cope with a maze of interactions.

Bugs in the brain's computer

One of my preparatory school teachers was an athletic disciplinarian as well as the school oracle. While the children in her class had a healthy respect for her effective follow-through with a rosewood hairbrush, they had less respect for her predictions. When she said it would rain, the sun shone.

Any politician she felt would win an election was doomed. When she was confident that we would win a football match we were certain to lose.

Her diagnosis of the cause of my stutter was one of her better efforts. She looked down my throat as though looking for a dislocated tonsil, shut my jaws with a neat snap, and said, 'It's just his nerves!'

Since all our actions, thoughts, and feelings are relayed by nerves, she couldn't be far wrong, and numerous scientists have tried to prove her right. A number of disabilities – for example, epilepsy, cluttering, and aphasia – are linked with abnormalities of the brain's nervous system caused by inheritance or injury. Many researchers have tried to link stuttering with brain structure and function, but most of them came up against the problem of distinguishing between cause and effect.

Although, as mentioned earlier, there is no solid evidence to support the long-held view that stuttering was caused by forcing left-handed children to use their right hands, the 'Cerebral Dominance Theory' was very popular in the 1920s and 1930s, and is being re-examined today. The theory was based on the assumption that normal speech occurs when one side (the left) of the cerebral cortex dominates the other (the right) for timing the nerve impulses controlling the muscles of those organs (lips, tongue, jaw, etc.) involved in speech. The supporters of the theory suggested that, if the left hemisphere is not sufficiently dominant, the co-ordination of the speech muscles will be poor, and the speech liable to break down. This theory lent credence to the idea that stuttering could be caused by forcing a left-handed child to become right-handed.

Like many other stutterers in the 1940s I sat with my head sprouting electrical terminals like a bionic man while some bright fellow watched the spikes on the chart of a machine trying to discover whether or not my brain waves were normal. Epileptics and people with brain damage have abnormal patterns, but mine seemed to be the common or garden, uninteresting type.

Nevertheless, studies in the 1940s produced evidence that,

compared to non-stutterers, some stutterers have a relatively high proportion of alpha rhythm (8 to 12 oscillations per second) in the cerebral cortex's left hemisphere. The stutterer's brain waves were sometimes out of phase if he was left-handed. [12]

One must realize, however, that the brain activity of a person who stutters is likely to be affected by the way he speaks; so that the problem of deciding what is cause and what is effect clouds the interpretation of these findings.

The early electroencephalographic (EEG) studies of stutterers were contradictory, partly because of rudimentary techniques. Modern research has demonstrated definite abnormalities in the cerebral cortex of some stutterers, but the relationships between these abnormalities and the predisposition to or the act of stuttering is far from clear.

Recent EEG studies by Einer Boberg, of the University of Alberta, Edmonton, and his colleagues at the Alberta Hospital in the same city support the view that stuttering is associated with abnormalities in the activity of the brain. Professor Boberg and his colleagues pointed out that, since Orton and Travis concluded in the 1920s that stutterers lacked the dominance of one side of the brain for speech functions, a great deal of evidence has been accumulated that people who stutter tend to lack the specialization of the left hemisphere of the brain that predominates in people with normal speech. [13] Quinn has suggested that people who stutter use the right hemisphere for speech and the left for non-verbal processing; [14] while other scientists have found that stutterers tend to process both speech and non-verbal activities in the right hemisphere, a reversal of the normal situation. [15]

Boberg and his colleagues examined the possibility that abnormal asymmetry of the brain's hemispheres was related to stuttering. They examined eleven stutterers, including two women, and measured their brain waves before and after three weeks of intensive speech therapy. In all cases the stutterers' speech improved, with two patients becoming almost totally fluent – at least in the clinic.

Before the speech therapy the stutterers showed abnormally high activity, during speech, in the posterior frontal region of the *right* hemisphere of the brain. After therapy the situation was reversed, the greatest activity being in the posterior frontal region of the *left* hemisphere of the brain.[16]

These findings indicate that treatment can shift the patterns of brain activity during speech from the 'abnormal' right to the 'normal' left. Once again, the problem of deciding what is cause and what is effect hovers in the background.

During a chat with one of the workers in this fascinating field I mentioned that I could write or draw mirror images with both hands simultaneously. His eyes lit up, and he cried, 'Aha! I know how your brain works!' I wish I did.

It was suggested that my right hemisphere may be unusually closely integrated with my left hemisphere. Because the billions of messages that cross my corpus callosum (the neurological telegraph line that links the two hemispheres) do so all too efficiently, the activity of my speech areas is mucked up. For years, I have consciously integrated my intuitive, creative, right-hemisphere activities with my logical left-hemisphere functions to boost my mental creativity. It worked remarkably well. I encouraged it, but maybe it made my stuttering worse. Anyway, I'm not going to change the habit. I'd rather stutter and be creative than be stutterless and lose those flashes of intuition and insight.

The muscle system, which is controlled by the motor tissues of the brain, has received a great deal of attention as a possible cause of stuttering. Control of the jaw muscles tends to be abnormal during stuttering, and it is well known that people who stutter have difficulty controlling their diaphragm, larynx, and breathing when they speak. Some feel that stutterers tend to lack co-ordination, but evidence is conflicting.[17] All of these differences are more likely to be the result of a person's struggle to speak rather than the cause of his disfluency.

One explanation was that stuttering is essentially a convulsion or muscular spasm similar to epilepsy: excitement, fear, and anxiety can trigger stuttering just as they do epilepsy. On this theory, stuttering is a series of small convulsions interfering with the speech.[18] Stuttering is sometimes associated with epilepsy, but there does not appear to be any strong, direct evidence to support this explanation.

The fact that stutterers find it difficult to move from one sound to the next gave rise to J. Eisenson's 'Perseveration Theory,' which attributes stuttering partly to an organic abnormality and partly to the stresses a stutterer is exposed to when he tries to speak.[19] Perseveration is simply the tendency for a pattern of behaviour to persevere. When it is applied to speech it refers to automatic and often involuntary abnormal continuation of speech behaviour. The stylus of your speech gets stuck in a rut.

According to this theory, when a stutterer speaks, the message or stimulus from the brain that orders the mind and muscles to adopt the conformation that produces a particular sound persists longer than is necessary. This prevents the speaker from moving to the next conformation needed for the next sound. The muscles switch on but do not switch off soon enough to permit fluency.

Eisenson proposed that people who stutter perseverate more than non-stutterers. He linked this constitutional or organic cause with the degree of meaning in the spoken words; the more meaningful the words, the more stutterers tend to stutter. He suggested that the temporary disruption of meaningful or propositional speech by perseveration could determine the degree of stuttering. He felt that only about 60 per cent of people who stutter perseverate for physical reasons; the others just perseverate (and stutter) according to the degree of significance they attach to their words and the difficulty of the speaking situation. These latter stutterers may not have a neurological problem.

Not all people who perseverate for physical reasons stutter. Some experts feel that the evidence supporting the theory is weak and that the relationships between the many factors involved are far from clear. Attempts to confirm the theory appear to have been unsuccessful, and at present the perseveration theory is not widely accepted. Nevertheless, the possibility of a link between physical and emotional origins of a stutter is interesting. Many stutterers, including myself, experience blocking in the middle of fluent speech with no change in situation and emotion, which makes them wonder if a physical switch turns off their fluency. It all serves to illustrate the difficulty of tracing a stutter to its source.

During the past two decades scientists trying to unravel the biology of the brain have created an information explosion. Melvin Konner, in his fascinating book *The Tangled Wing: Biological Constraints on the Human Spirit*,[20] describes how brain activity affects our feelings of fear, joy, grief, lust, and love, and how new knowledge and techniques are providing fresh insights into human behaviour. It is possible that new information will help us determine whether a child is physically predisposed to stutter. Recent investigations of brain abnormalities associated with dyslexia, a disorder of perception and communication, raise many questions.

The parallel of dyslexia

Dyslexia interferes with a person's ability to read, write, and spell. Not surprisingly, this makes learning difficult. Dyslexics vary in their symptoms, but most of them distort words and sentences and have difficulty distinguishing letters with similar shapes. They may have trouble writing down words they hear, may confuse left and right, may reverse series of numbers in calculations, and may even have difficulty pronouncing words.

Although dyslexia is very different from a stutter, there are striking parallels with stuttering. For example more boys than girls are dyslexic; the handicap seems to run in families; many dyslexics are left-handed or ambidextrous; the disability appears to be unpredictable, with the dyslexic being able to read correctly on some occasions and not on others; dyslexics' IQs are more or less normal; society (including impatient, uninformed parents and teachers) tends to label dyslexics as stupid or mentally retarded and to taunt and penalize them; and many dyslexics suffer from low self-esteem. All of these apply to stutterers. Even the early research on stuttering, with its emphasis on dominance of the brain's hemispheres, genetics, neuroses, and environmental pressures, parallels early research on dyslexia. Dyslexia, as with stuttering, is treated by teaching the patient how to control and live with his handicap rather than how to cure it. Both dyslexia and stuttering take a great deal of skill and effort to control because both involve many interacting factors.

Recent studies of the brains of dyslexics indicate that the handicap may be associated with abnormal patterns in the nerve cells in the 'speech zone' of the brain's left cerebral hemisphere. The evidence is still incomplete and the conclusions tentative, but the fact that the brains of some foetuses show similar aberrations suggests an early breakdown in the patterns of brain development, possibly caused by abnormal hormone levels.[21]

As with stutterers, early studies of dyslexics' brains revealed no abnormalities, but new techniques may show otherwise. What if both dyslexia and stuttering prove to be neurological disorders? Will this mean they can be treated more easily? Not necessarily; but it may at least permit early diagnosis and treatment before the handicaps produce emotional problems that are difficult to deal with in later life. If it turns out that stuttering and dyslexia are caused by abnormal neurotransmitter gradients, then medication could also be helpful. For the time being, we must wait and see what the scientists come up with next. The pendulum seems to be swinging again toward hypotheses of organic origins for stutters, after a long period of disfavour.

Whatever science uncovers, my school teacher was right. It's just nerves.

Stuttering and sound

The railway engines of my childhood were magnificent, smelly monsters that rumbled like flatulent elephants, hissed white clouds of steam, and belched volcanoes of grey, gritty smoke. On their black, gleaming sides they sported polished brass name plates with aristocratic titles like *The Duke of York*. They were quite different from the diesels that throb quietly along our modern tracks like faceless bureaucrats. When three or four of the old, noisy beasts were in a railway station and thunderous rumbles hammered at my ears, I was perfectly fluent.

Years later in the Armed Forces I welcomed the shattering roar when we warmed up the Rolls-Royce Merlin Spitfire engines during morning check-up. Nobody suggested that we should wear earguards, so, as one fitter said, we couldn't hear ourselves think. Every day for this short period I was fluent. Even though I had to shout to make myself understood, the respite from the stress of trying to speak was welcome.

The majority of people who stutter can speak more fluently when they can't hear themselves. Very few deaf people stutter. In my case I wasn't sure if the fluency was because I couldn't hear myself or because I had to shout, because stutterers are often more fluent when they speak loudly. During timber cruises I had no difficulty calling tree measurements to the record keeper. Speech pathologists share this uncertainty about what causes the fluency in noisy situations, but it seems that blocking out stutterers' lower speech frequencies by noise increases fluency whether they speak loudly or not.[22]

The effect of noise on fluency has led to a number of theories. Some scientists hold the view that noise is just a distraction; others feel that noise affects the perception of speech feedback. All people with normal hearing hear themselves speak and automatically monitor what they have said. The theory is that there is a delay in the feedback from a stutterer's speech caused by an organic difference in the hearing process.

The level of noise seems to be important. Ninety decibels produce almost normal fluency, 50 decibels reduce disfluency, and below 50 decibels there is little effect. Lower frequencies (less than 500 Hz) appear to be most effective in producing fluency, and this has been used in therapy.

The obvious inference is that the stutterer's response to sounds differs from the non-stutterer's. There is evidence that stutterers differ from non-stutterers in their perception of sound, but only at frequencies of 2,000 Hz, which is puzzling.[23] Another inference could be that since boys are more likely to stutter than girls, boys should differ from girls in their feedback of speech. A study of eight male and eight female non-stutterers showed that when the speech feedback was artificially delayed by about 0.2 to 0.8 second, the males developed speech patterns similar to a stutter, and the females did not. There is some doubt that this artificial stutter is the same as a real stutter, but females may deal with speech perception in a different way from males.

When the feedback of speech is delayed by about 0.2 second and amplified, the speech of normal speakers tends to disintegrate. [24] When stutterers are exposed to this delayed auditory feedback (DAF), the speech of the more severe stutterers tends to improve, while others have the same difficulty as non-stutterers. [25]

Some scientists feel that the effects of noise on fluency indicate that stuttering is a perceptual rather than a motor disorder. Shane suggested that noise removed the anxiety of people who stutter by obliterating their perception of their own stuttering. [26] Many experts still feel that sound helps the stutterer mainly because it is distracting.

There are still many questions to be answered. Do all stutterers respond to noise in the same way? Does the benefit fade when the novelty of noise wears off? Can some stutterers still perceive their speech in spite of noise and yet remain fluent? Is the frequency of a sound all that important?

Whenever somebody comes up with an idea of how something works, an engineer is sure to get in on the act. Stuttering is no exception. A great many of our bodily functions involve servomechanisms or automatic controls. When we get hot, the body's thermostat automatically controls our temperature (unless we are sick); when we run up a steep hill the body's controls stimulate the cardiovascular system to pump more oxygen to our flagging tissues; and when we are afraid, adrenalin is fed into the bloodstream to help us handle the situation. We possess sensor units that respond to our body's signals and send information to the controller units that compare what we need with what we have. If there is a deficiency or a surplus, a controller signals to the gland or tissue concerned to do something about it.

Normal speech appears to be an automatic process, regulated by feedback from many sources and involving a servomechanism with automatic controls. The ear acts as the sensor and hears the voice production from the vocal machinery. The controller, with its ability to compare what we want to say with what we have said, is somewhere in the brain. If what we have said does not complete what we want to say, an error signal goes out for the body to complete the communication. [27]

This feedback theory of speech was linked with the discovery that many stutterers become more fluent when the feedback of their speech to the ear's sensor is masked. The theory is that stuttering is a breakdown in the speech's automatic controls. The breakdown is caused by disruption of the feedback circuits that integrate thought and speech, or by responses to false error signals that arise from anticipated problems with fluency. Stuttering could also be caused by a fault in the sensor unit (conduction of sound to the ear), or by negative feedback from a listener ('I don't understand. Please repeat.'), which prompts the child to develop the habit of repeating himself.[28] — Bloodstein

Cybernetic models like this are useful because they encourage the scientist to organize his thoughts in a logical manner, provide insights into interactions between speech components, and help the researcher to ask the right questions. They may not produce specific answers, but they do provide a valuable framework. The approach, which takes into account possible physical abnormalities as well as effects of feedback from listeners or from anticipated difficulty (anxiety), also, refreshingly, breaks down the artificial distinctions between organic and non-organic causes of stutters.

The effects on stuttering of delayed auditory feedback and masking with low-frequency noise are still the subject of debate. They are just two of the keys to the prison of a stutter, with its numerous locks and alarms.

Stutterers' physiology

The concept of human biorhythms is based on the fact that everyone's levels of vitality, clearness of thought, and co-ordination vary from day to day. Since ancient times people have believed that the phases of the moon affect mental activity, with werewolves, vampires, and other mythical nasties carrying out their dirty deeds when the moon is full. There are many who feel that atmospheric pressure affects mood; and, indeed, a succession of grey, rainy days does make me sluggish and irritable. Any change in mood, vitality, or co-ordination can affect the fluency of a stutterer. On those days when I wake with a brain that feels like cold rice pudding, clumsy fingers that drop the breakfast cereal packet, and a lack of concentration that makes me burn the bacon, my words seem to wade ankle deep in molasses. As Van Riper wrote, my mode of speech is gluency rather than fluency.

All of these daily changes are the result of shifts in our physiological processes. In spite of the fact that scientists have not found any clear physiological differences between stutterers and non-stutterers, completely to divorce stuttering from physiology would be absurd. Although the experimental results are inconclusive, it is useful to examine them, particularly those of relevance to therapy. All people who stutter hope that one day some genius will find out that stuttering is caused by a biochemical deficiency that can be cured by a magic pill, making unnecessary all the hard work and frustration of extended speech therapy. It doesn't seem likely that the complex syndrome of stuttering will respond to such simple treatment, but we can hope.

The trouble with studying the physiology of stuttering is that both stuttering and expecting to stutter cause physiological changes arising from associated stress and anxiety. This state can persist for some time after speaking – basically, until the speaker's frustration diminishes. When a silent stutterer is being studied by a scientist, the stutterer's attention is focused on his quiescent speech and he is likely to be nervous even when silent. Some scientists have been careful to allow for this and others have not, so results need to be scrutinized carefully.

Several early studies suggested that a stutterer's heartbeat is faster than a non-stutterer's; but other studies have indicated otherwise.[29] Even in carefully controlled conditions, stutterers had more variations in heart rate and faster heartbeats than others, and there were suggestions of sex differences. The pulse rate of females with normal speech tends to be faster than that of males; but, when the pulses of young male and female stutterers were examined, the opposite was true.[30] Other workers found that, although females usually have lower basal metabolic rates than males, these rates were relatively high in female stutterers.[31] The research results were interpreted by some scientists to mean that stuttering was associated with differences in metabolism and sex, but nobody was rash enough to use the word 'cause.' These conclusions were based on shaky experimental grounds and are not widely accepted. The vocal tension of a person who stutters is obvious. This led to the study of voice mechanisms, particularly the behaviour of the larynx, which was admirably reviewed by C. Woodruff Starkweather.[32] It is hard to sort out cause and effect, and research has been inconclusive.

Other studies have shown that, compared to non-stutterers, people who stutter have high levels of blood sugar, calcium, phosphorus, albumen, and globulin, high urinary creatinine, and a greater tendency to allergies, but later evidence has contradicted this.[33]

Because a person who stutters can get quite worked up about the act of speaking, you'd expect scientists to have looked at blood pressures carefully. However, there is remarkably little information in the literature on the subject. Early studies of the blood pressures of male stutterers and non-stutterers indicated that there were no differences, but later evidence suggests that a male stutterer's blood pressure increases when he tries to speak, which is to be expected.[34]

The reported high carbon-dioxide content of the stutterer's blood became the basis of a carbon-dioxide therapy that was popular for a few years.[35] The idea was that the relatively high acidity of the stutterer's blood was caused by high levels of carbon dioxide, although some scientists didn't agree. In spite of the doubts, carbon-dioxide gas was administered to thirty-three stutterers. A third of them (eleven) became much more fluent; others (twelve) showed a little improvement; and the rest did not respond at all. Other attempts were made to use carbon dioxide, sometimes with nitrous-oxide gas, but success was variable. Stutterers whose impediment began in adolescence or later seemed to respond better to carbon dioxide than stutterers who developed their problem when very young. The usefulness of carbon-dioxide therapy and the implications of carbon-dioxide levels in the blood are very much in doubt.[36]

Several attempts were also made to link stutters with endocrine malfunction. It was known in 1928 that when some non-stuttering patients were given a thyroid extract they started to stutter, and that the stuttering stopped when the dose ceased. Unfortunately, the recorded stuttering could have been cluttering, a different disorder, since cluttering can develop when thyroid extracts are administered.[37]

There are many physiological differences between stutterers and non-stutterers, but not one is beyond dispute or can be labelled as the cause of a stutter. People who stutter are notoriously hard to study in an objective way. All results tend to be clouded by physiological changes associated with the approach to speaking, the moment of stuttering, and its aftermath.

Anticipation, anxiety, conflicts, and cues

You never get used to a stutter no matter how long you have it. Those people who say they don't care are kidding themselves. Any stutterer who is honest with himself will admit that he feels a chilling fear whenever he anticipates speaking at length in front of a large audience. There are public speakers with severe stutters who manage to cope, and I asked one of them how he felt about blocking and grimacing in front of a large number of people. His reply was, 'It doesn't really bother me,' and he obviously believed it. He must have learned to anaesthetize his feelings so well that if he did care he didn't realize it. My next question was whether he found public speaking stressful and exhausting. He said, 'No, of course not,' but his eyes said the opposite.

Anticipation of stuttering can be unnerving, and there have been many times when I've wanted to take to the hills (and a few times when I have). The more you fear that your speech will break down, the worse the stutter becomes. It is not surprising that speech pathologists have looked closely at the effects of fearful anticipation on fluency. Their work was the basis of the 'Anticipatory Struggle Theory,' which, in spite of the fact that it is based on many intangibles, makes a great deal of sense to many stutterers, who find it seems to fit their disability.[38]

The hypothesis proposes that a person who stutters interferes with his own speech (i.e., stutters) because he believes, either consciously or unconsciously, that speaking is difficult. The stutterer becomes disfluent when he anticipates that he is going to stutter, which on the surface seems to be a chicken-or-egg situation. It can be argued that if he didn't stutter he wouldn't anticipate stuttering, and, consequently, that fearful anticipation can't be the cause of a stutter. This riddle is resolved when it is realized that speech experts distinguish between the factors affecting the *onset* of a stutter (i.e., its early beginnings) and the factors affecting the speech at or immediately before the *moment* of stuttering. A child may begin to stutter for one or more of the reasons discussed earlier in this chapter (neurosis, brain malfunction, auditory feedback, parental and social pressures, etc.); but the future development of the childish, hesitant stutter into a major, well-established stutter is affected by the memory of speech failure, with all its attendant humiliation, rejection, and frustration, and the anxiety that it will happen again. It is hard to allay such fears.

Many emotions and situations affect the fluency of an established stutterer, and anxiety plays a major role. If a person for many years experiences a sharp pain when he bends over, he will be a bit nervous and careful about bending – with good reason. Similarly, the stutterer has good reason to worry about speaking. He knows from experience that whenever he speaks it is highly likely that he will block, stutter, grimace, and get a bad response from his audience. He anticipates that he will struggle to speak. So he struggles and stutters.

The hypothesis involves the idea that a stutterer doesn't stutter if he doesn't think about his speech. If you think too hard about what you are doing and don't trust your automatic reflexes, you are likely to make a mess of anything, whether you are playing the piano, walking a tightrope, or doing the pole-vault.

I once climbed a razor-backed ridge with drops of a thousand feet or so on both sides. It was no great feat. The well-worn track was a yard wide, my boots were cleated, and I don't suffer from vertigo. I happily plodded upwards bouncing echoes off the black cliffs for fun until I came to a metal plaque in memory of someone who had stepped into the void. It made me more careful. Thereafter I watched my feet, assessed the chances of my cleats' skidding on the veins of hard quartz, and made sure that my centre of gravity didn't stray too far to one side or the other. To my dismay, I began to stumble and scrabble, and a flicker of apprehension soon blossomed into a sickening fear. The chasms looked horrifying and, for the first time, I froze on a mountain. I sat on a rock, ate some chocolate, calmed down, and reminded myself that, since my feet knew their job, I'd better let them get on with it. I switched onto automatic and contentedly bounced echoes all the way to the top.

Speech can be like that. When you think about all the lip, tongue, larynx, and word co-ordination involved you are liable to fall into the abyss of disfluency. Anybody with the tendency to stutter may well freeze from fear of speaking. The old story about the centipede who was crippled when ordered to explain how it walked has been refined by scientists who contend that the stutterer gets into trouble when he consciously tries to produce and synchronize all of the speech movements instead of relying on his automatic co-ordination.

Early students of stuttering were aware of the fears and doubts associated with disfluency and suggested that the impediment could be caused by faulty auto-suggestion, or a deep-seated neurotic conviction of speech failure, or the lack of automatic speech mentioned earlier.[39]

The anticipated struggle involves a large element of avoidance. Wendell Johnson and his colleagues felt that stuttering is an attempt to avoid an anticipated, feared breakdown of fluency. Rather than being caused by neuroses and brain abnormalities, it is a disorder of perception precipitated by society and its demands for verbal communication.[40] In this kind of situation stutterers are damned if they try to avoid stuttering and damned if they stutter. It's not surprising that some of them lapse into silence. They want to speak but at the same time don't want to speak. This conflict has led to the idea that stuttering results from the desire to avoid speech. Avoidance and anxiety rear their ugly heads again. The 'Approach-Avoidance Conflict Theory' developed by J.G. Sheehan is used a great deal in therapy. It differs a little from the idea of stuttering to avoid stuttering in that it implies that a person stutters to avoid speaking.[41]

Sheehan's theory also involves the idea that when a stutterer blocks, his block actually reduces his fear. In other words, much of the fear felt by a stutterer arises from an attempt to hide from his audience the fact that he stutters. When he blocks there is no need to try and hide the stutter. It is obvious to everybody that his speech has broken down. Consequently the fear associated with hiding the disfluency is reduced. Stutterers can put enormous emotional effort into hiding their stutters by switching roles and changing words. Teaching a stutterer to stop changing words is an important part of therapy.

Another facet of the anticipatory struggle theory is the 'preparatory set' developed by Charles Van Riper in the United States. That is, as the stutterer approaches a feared word, he directs his attention onto his speech organs and tensely approaches the word. He prepares for the first difficult sound with a fixed speaking posture and may even rehearse the dreaded sound, making it impossible for him to say the word normally. He approaches the word with a prepared set of muscular and psychological positions, and, as happened to me on the mountain, he stumbles.[42]

Oliver Bloodstein summarized the complex anticipatory struggle theory as a sequence. First there is a suggestion that speaking is difficult. Failure is therefore expected, and a need to avoid failure is felt. Normal automatic speech is replaced by a short-term speaking strategy. The physical and mental sets to carry out the strategy are mustered, and the result is tension and fragmented speech.[43]

During the early 1970s I found myself involved in work that required a great deal of telephoning. Although many of the numbers were on automatic dialling, I often had to request extension numbers or give my own number. Every time I asked for or gave a number I scanned digits looking for road blocks. 'Nine' was a nightmare; I would either block or 'nnnn' like a hornet. 'Two' was tricky, but not so bad. On 'six' and 'seven' I was liable to hiss like a viper, and on 'four' or 'five' my 'fffff' sounded like a slow puncture. 'Three' was fine and only tied my tongue in a knot occasionally. 'Eight' and 'zero' always slid out on well-oiled wheels. My own number was 589-2880. I slow-punctured my way through 'five,' blocked on 'nine' and 'two,' and breezed by the 'eights' and 'zero.' French numerals were terrible. Only *'un'* and *'huit'* stood a fair chance of coming out of my mouth untangled. I could easily predict on which sounds my speech would freeze. Stutterers are remarkably good at forecasting their troubles.

Stutterers' forecasts of speech blockages were found to be between 85 and 96 per cent correct. According to the anticipatory struggle theory, stutterers are not clairvoyant, but simply stutter when they expect to do so.[44]

The participants in these experiments were well aware of the speech blocks ahead, but conscious anticipation of stuttering does not inevitably fragment the speech. Many stutterers I know sometimes block completely on words they can usually say fluently. I do the same and, even during a phase of complete fluency when I am thinking about my research more than my speech, I can suddenly come to a dead halt, much to my surprise. I used to think that a neurological circuit had shorted out, but it may be that the anticipation of blocks is unconscious or subliminal, conditioned by past experience.

All of us, whether we have normal speech or stutter, suffer from delusions about our fluency. Normal speakers are usually unaware of their normal disfluencies and get quite a shock when they hear themselves on a tape recorder ('Is that me ...?'). I sometimes think that I have been fluent when in fact I blocked in a minor way about ten times each minute. I tend to notice the major, debilitating blocks and don't register the minor hesitations and repetitions.

I know very well that speaking to an audience of fifteen is harder for me than to an audience of four, and this has nothing to do with conventional stage fright. Standing and talking to a mike at a lecture is harder than talking when I sit in a chair. I am much more fluent when I can see my audience – that's why I never speak and show colour transparencies at the same time, and why the telephone is so difficult.

One of the speaking situations I try to forget occurred when I had just taken on a new job in Oxford. Within the first month I was told to visit the Meteorological Office. I was a little nervous about my speech. I anticipated trouble, and I got it! I was marched straight into an auditorium and asked to tell an audience of about fifty scientists and managers about my work. I started to block badly and nearly took to my heels, but controlled myself and called upon my personal wily devil that gets me out of that kind of mess. I changed my tactics and told them that I was new to the job and was there to ask them questions – which I did, stutter and all. It went very well. They did most of the talking.

The trouble with going to fortune tellers is that they might tell you something bad is going to happen, and that they might be right. Stutterers see their own speech future remarkably clearly. It is usually bad, and their predictions are nearly always right on the nail.

Although a stutterer can predict most of the sounds and some of the situations that will provoke his stutter, he finds it difficult to understand what triggers bad speech phases. He is bewildered when his speech collapses around him for no reason that he can perceive. Some scientists feel that the occurrence of stuttering, once it is firmly established, is fairly consistent and can be triggered by definite learned cues. This, of course, refers to events that precipitate the moment of stuttering after the impediment is established, not to the onset of disfluency in childhood. The alleged causes of the onset and of the moment of stuttering may be quite different.

It was noticed by Wendell Johnson and his co-workers that, when stutterers read a passage several times, the number of hesitations tended to decrease because they adapted to the situation, but the places on the page where a patient blocked were always more or less the same. About 65 per cent of the words stuttered in one reading were stuttered in the next. Either the position of the words or their meaning precipitated the blocks. Stuttering is not haphazard, whatever the bewildered stutterer may think.[45]

Several stutterers were tested to find out whether their memories of past difficult words cued further speech difficulty. All the subjects read a passage, and the words upon which they stuttered were blanked out on the script. They read the passage again, and, as before, the stuttered words were blanked out. This was repeated several times until most of the stuttering was removed. The few remaining stuttered words were next to blocked-out words that had given the stutterer difficulty in previous readings, so the stutterers appeared to respond to cues of past failure (the nearby blocked-out words) rather than to the form or meaning of the words. If the stuttered words were removed from the page and the text closed up to fill the gaps, stuttering was much less than when the blocked-out words remained on the page. People who stutter seem to respond to cues related to past difficulties.[46]

This led to the theory that the moment of stuttering involves a cue that evokes anticipation of trouble, and that this results in attempts to avoid stuttering. Of course, this fits in well with the idea of anticipated struggle. The struggle is the stutter. The cues may not even be words. Colours and light intervals associated with past stuttering have been used in experiments to condition stutterers to be more disfluent.[47]

Why I stuttered more on one word than another was a mystery until I read about Spencer Brown's research in the 1930s and early 1940s.

Brown found that in thirty-two adults with stutters, about 90 per cent of their stuttering was on the first sounds of words, and the rest of the hesitations were on sounds at the beginning of syllables, particularly the accented syllables in long words. Brown also observed that while the likelihood of stuttering was affected by the sounds of the words, this varied a great deal from one stutterer to another. Most of his subjects, however, stuttered more on consonants than on vowels. This may have been caused by the fact that consonants are more important in communication (some languages don't have vowels), by the greater tension of lip and tongue, by the interruption of air flow, or simply by the fact that there are more consonants than vowels.[48]

The sound doesn't appear to be completely responsible for triggering the stutter. Words starting with 'f' give me more trouble than those beginning with 'ph,' and 'ph' is easier for me than the plosive 'p,' which seems illogical. Bloodstein quotes the case of the New York City boy who, when he read aloud, blocked on words starting with 'th' and had no difficulty with 't' and 'd' in spite of the fact that with his accent he pronounced 'th' as 't' or 'd,' as in 'tink' and 'dis.' This sounds absurd until the principles of anticipated avoidance are applied. The 'th' cued anticipated failure, the stutterer tried to avoid disfluency, struggled, and blocked. The phonetics were secondary.[49]

Although many stuttering children have trouble with pronouns and conjunctions, when adults read aloud they stutter more on nouns, verbs, adjectives, and adverbs than on pronouns, conjunctions, articles, and prepositions. This suggests that the main problems are associated with the words that contain the most information. You can shorten the sentence 'The red cat sat on the woolly blue mat' to 'Red cat sat woolly blue mat' without losing much meaning. People who stutter get into trouble on important words. What could be more loaded than: 'John Smith; born 2 February 1934; Residence, 2 Maple Street, Felixville, Ontario; Telephone number: 613-576-2112.' No wonder a stutterer, faced by a battery of loaded nouns, falls apart when asked to give his basic data.

I am often fluent after a few blocks and repetitions in the first sentence or so. Like a car engine started at thirty below, my speech motor warms up – but it can conk out later, like a car when the gas line freezes. Brown found that stutterers have more trouble with the first and early words in sentences than with later words. I always find that the first words in a sentence look like a crag to be climbed as I prepare to relinquish anxiety-free silence for anxiety-loaded speech. Scientists feel that the conspicuousness of the early words are the stutterer's downfall, fitting in with the idea of anticipated struggle. The crag looms up, the struggle to climb it is anticipated, the struggle begins, and the speech falls apart.

I've always been nervous about long, hyphenated words with their double or even triple barrels pointing at my speech, making me all too conscious of my speech anxiety's hair trigger. Stutterers in general have more trouble with long words than short ones, possibly because it is harder to say them, or possibly because they stand out in the sentence.[50] Anything that looks hard to say to a stutterer is likely to give him trouble.

In order to simplify this tangled web of influences, Oliver Bloodstein summarized the conditions that appear to affect a stutterer's sometime fluency (as when singing, reciting, whispering, speaking in unison, or acting another role) or lack of fluency (as when talking to other people). Rather than seek the fundamental causes that precipitated the stutter in childhood, he concentrated on why the fluency of an established stutterer varies to such a large extent.

He supplemented the results of other workers with a survey of his own, in which he solicited views on the conditions affecting the fluency of young adults, and was able to define 115 situations that affected the stutter.[51] There was considerable variation from one individual to another according to the different meanings the situations had for each person. When asked 'Do you stutter when speaking to a parent?' the response would depend on whether or not the parent was supportive or antagonistic about the impediment. After allowing for such variables, Bloodstein was able to recognize the following eight broad classes of factors that either increased or decreased stuttering:

1 Communication content
2 Listener's reaction
3 Desire for approval
4 Distractions
5 Response to suggestion
6 Changes in physical tension
7 Period between planning to speak and speaking
8 Presence or absence of stuttering cues

The *communication content* of words plays an important role in stuttering. A person who stutters does so more when reading passages that have meaning than when reading meaningless words. He can usually sing, count, read in unison, shadow other speakers, swear, recite, talk to a dog, tease a baby, read lists that the audience can see, engage in banal social chit-chat at parties, and say 'Hello,' 'Goodbye,' 'Thank you,' and 'Have a nice day.' He can be fluent when he says anything that doesn't contain much meaning or involve the responsibility of communicating.

I even stuttered talking to my dog. He was very bright, understood many words, and seemed to know what I was saying. My experience with tape recording is a good example of the effect of meaningful communication on fluency. When I worked for the government I had sufficient speech control to make recordings with no effort at all when the only person who heard them later was myself. Nevertheless, when I dictated a letter to my secretary on the tape recorder, I had to use learned speaking techniques very carefully indeed or I soon lost control. It was the same audience – the tape recorder – but the communication content (and context) of the dictation differed.

I can say tongue-twisters quickly and fluently, so there's nothing wrong with my muscular co-ordination. My motor system and my brain's speech centres seem to fire on all their cylinders. Ask me to *describe* the phonetics of the tongue-twister, however, and I'm soon floundering in the quicksands of disfluency.

The *listener's reaction* plays another key role. I can usually tell whether a stranger and I are going to get along within a minute of meeting him. Even seeing photographs of certain types of people can jolt the stability of my speech. (Many others have found this, too.)[52] It seems to be a matter of the cues described earlier in this chapter. The speech can be disrupted by a particular type of person or even by a cue associated with the person. In general, when the listener shows (or seems to show, because people who stutter sometimes see reactions that aren't there) embarrassment, impatience, shock, hostility, amusement, or pity, a confirmed stutterer's fluency often scatters to the four winds. He may be completely fluent with a friend who sees him daily and is familiar with his strange way of speaking.

People who stutter tend to be visually acute, sometimes too acute for their own peace of mind. They seem to pick up vibes remarkably well. Even when well hidden, a person's surprise at hearing me stutter can affect my speech.

While some stutterers find it easy to talk at home, others find that their worst speaking situation. Many adolescents I have spoken to found that their parents' lack of sympathy about their stutter made it worse (a two-way street if one of the parents also stutters!). Audience reaction is important and may be one reason I find it hard to speak to audiences of more than five or six; the larger the audience, the more likely it is that some of them will respond badly to my hesitations. I used to describe listener response as audience interaction, because I would respond to the audience myself, quite apart from stuttering; in turn, my response would affect their response, and so on.

Desire for approval affects stutterers in many ways, and many need approval to keep fluent. Others, like myself, find out early in life that when a person stutters approval comes his way in small doses. These people learn to survive with very little. You have to speak and you know that people will react badly, so you tend to say 'To hell with it!' and get on with communicating, letting the audience think what they wish.

People who stutter are inclined to have trouble speaking to those in positions of authority, particularly when such individuals are formally dressed.[53] Conversely, a stutterer is often more fluent when he *is* the person in authority and is speaking to subordinates. Stutterers vary, though, and this didn't work in my case. I was relatively fluent talking to superiors (sometimes more fluent than they liked), and my stutter became worse as I rose in the government's scientific hierarchy and talked to more subordinates, probably because of increasing administrative frustration.

The idea that leaders stutter less when talking to the led didn't work for me in my school's Officers' Training Corps, either. I was fluently drilling a platoon when I blocked badly on the word 'Halt!' My soldiers determinedly marched straight into a wooden pavilion and ended up in a laughing heap of tangled arms, legs, and Lee-Enfield rifles.

The fluency of a male stutterer's conversation with a female, and vice versa, depends a great deal on approval. A pretty girl who feels that boys approve of her appearance may be more fluent in a girl-boy situation than when talking to girls. Some males who stutter, fearing and often getting rejection by girls, may well be more disfluent in boy-girl conversations. I never had much trouble talking to girls, although I had my fair share of 'Get lost.' Since I was educated in one of those monastic boys' schools where the boys don't talk to a girl for months on end, and spent years enthusiastically repairing the omission, I was spared the nastiness that adolescent girls show to white blackbirds in the flock.

Distractions that divert a stutterer's attention away from his fear of disfluency, his stuttering cues, the information content of his words, and the response of listeners are likely to help him to control his speech. The stronger the distraction, the greater the control. This has been the basis of several therapies, most of which help for only a short time. Any exposure to unusually stimulating situations tends to increase fluency. It is safe to guess that few people who stutter have major speech problems on their honeymoons.

Bloodstein wrote that 'speaking in a monotone, whispering, shouting, using an abnormally high pitch or an abnormally low pitch, adopting an unusual voice quality, speaking with exaggerated articulatory movements, or with slurred articulation, with objects in the mouth, at a slow rate, with altered breathing, or in time to rhythmical movements' all tend to improve fluency.[54] These all distract the speaker.

When I was about nine years old I heard that objects held in the mouth increased the fluency of people with tangled tongues. What could be more sensible than to experiment with one of my most treasured glass marbles, a large, opaque, blue-and-red beauty called a 'Mex,' which was worth ten transparent marbles in the school market. I popped it into my mouth and spoke fluently to a sceptical friend who unfortunately cracked a joke about losing my marbles. I laughed, choked, and swallowed my Mex so that it was necessary for me to stay in hospital on a diet of dry bread and sips of water until my Mex reappeared. It was gratifying to find that in subsequent games my Mex had increased in value by 300 per cent after its long and mysterious journey. I still have it.

A stuttering colleague of mine used the slurred speech technique with remarkable success, even on public platforms. Unfortunately it gave the wrong impression and he was approached on several occasions by advocates of Alcoholics Anonymous.

Any distraction seems to help a stutterer for a while, and dancing, piano-playing, swimming, and operating a machine have been cited as examples. I haven't tried swimming and talking at the same time, but it sure would focus my attention on timing my breathing.

The idea of *response to suggestion*, hypnotic or otherwise, has always fascinated stutterers, who have a mental image of a wise, old man swinging a shiny disc on a chain before their eyes and lulling them into a deep sleep from which they emerge completely fluent. This is, of course, wishful thinking. I do not hypnotize easily. The only time anybody succeeded, he cured me of hayfever instead of my stutter – which raised a few eyebrows among professional immunologists. Nevertheless, some stutterers respond to suggesions that they need not worry about their hesitations and become fluent for short periods. For example, a Frenchman used non-hypnotic powers of suggestion so effectively that a stutterer's fluency improved for a week until his speech collapsed to a state worse than before.[55] Stutterers, like most people, can be brainwashed to do a great many things, but suggesting that they speak fluently seems to be a little too much. It may help some people, but there are dangers, unless the treatment is handled with great care.

It has always been said that *changes in physical tension* affect the severity of a stutter. I have tried many relaxation tapes and auto-suggestion techniques that were supposed to relax me, but they had no effect at all. A great many stutterers feel that relaxation of physical tension helps their fluency and that they stutter more when scared or stressed, but the effect on fluency of physical relaxation seems to vary from one person to another. I have always wondered how you can relax deeply and expose yourself to tension-filled stuttering cues and bad stuttering situations at the same time. If somebody could have taught me how to relax my anxiety about speaking, that would have been much more useful.

The *period between planning to speak and speaking* used to have devastating effects on my speech until I achieved better control. Fortunately my surname begins with 'C', so my sojourn in purgatory before descending into the hell of having to read aloud in class was mercifully short.

Later in life I had terrible problems at round-table committee meetings of thirty or forty people when each participant had to stand up in turn and introduce himself. Not only were my name, position, organization, and occupation hard for a person with my kind of stutter to say, but the delay in saying it seemed to be interminable, and my anxiety mounted exponentially. Since the final result was always a disaster, I preferred to chair and control the meetings myself, or to arrive five minutes late.

The tendency for stutterers' speech to fall apart when they are forced to wait for periods as short as ten seconds before speaking has been confirmed experimentally.[56] Delays of three minutes used to bring me out in goose-bumps of apprehension. If I have to make a mess of something, I like to get it over with.

The eighth situation affecting fluency – *the presence or absence of stuttering cues* (e.g., the grammatical identity of words, their position in the sentence, their meaning and phonetics, the type of situation, and the response of the listener) – spills over into the other seven situations of Bloodstein's list. As he points out, the greater the number of these cues in the situation, the more chance there is that the stutterer's speech will fall apart.

Some cues can be removed by changing a stutterer's location, at least for a while. One stutterer was a virtual nomad. He stayed in a place until his speech deteriorated and then moved on.

Bloodstein's eight categories usefully organize the many factors affecting an established stutterer's speech and the paradoxes associated with it. As he says, all of these categories essentially boil down to anxiety about stuttering.

Although Bloodstein's categories refer mainly to the moment of stuttering associated with an established impediment, few will deny that anxiety about communication pervades a child's speech behaviour once he is conscious that he is different from others. All stutterers are anxious about their speech; those who deny it are either not aware of their anxieties or are not prepared to admit them.

Some speech pathologists do not accept these complex ideas about stuttering. They feel that, no matter what caused the stutter, most people with stutters just speak the wrong way and can be retrained to speak correctly – that there is no need to treat the whole person and his anxieties. R.L. Webster developed his program of fluency modification because he felt that so many of the theoretical notions about stuttering are 'cumbersome' and 'poorly defined.'[57]

The role of anxiety, word fear, and stuttering cues cannot be ignored, but neither can the more direct behavioural approaches. The answer probably lies between the two, and a great deal of good modern therapy uses both approaches in combinations best suited to individuals.

The impact of these ideas on therapy will be discussed in the next chapter. The stuttering syndrome and the human psyche are so complex that it is not surprising that stuttering is difficult to control. What is surprising is the amount of success speech pathologists have under the circumstances.

FIVE

How do you treat stuttering?

'There are no such things as incurables; there are only things for which man has not found a cure.'

Bernard M. Baruch

A few years ago I accidentally overheard one of our executives (a man noted more for his loud voice than for his tact; the kind of overbearing person who thinks that if you say something loudly enough and often enough it must be true) talking about me. He said, in a voice everybody in the building could hear, 'You'd think Carlisle would do something about that darned stuttering! If he made the effort he could speak as well as I can. I knew a kid who cured his stutter by the age of thirteen. You'd think an adult like Carlisle would make the effort.'

No doubt he heard my loud and scatological response (the walls were thin), because the conversation abruptly ceased. Nevertheless, he reflected the commonly held view that stuttering is easy to cure if the individual makes the effort. People can always cite examples of someone they know who overcame the disability when young. 'If one person can do it, why can't they all do it?' is the feeling.

Most people ignore the fact that stuttering varies from person to person. Many slight stutters spontaneously disappear in early childhood or adolescence for reasons that are not fully understood. Some stutterers are relatively easy to treat. Nevertheless, when a severe stutter persists in an adult, it is usually the self-reinforcing kind, where disfluency breeds anxiety and tension, which in turn make the stuttering worse, which creates still more stress, and so on. This type is usually difficult to treat, and cures are rare.

Responsible therapists treating adults with severe stutters don't promise a cure. They can help the adult stutterer get better control, reduce the silent, stressful blocks, improve fluency, and reduce anxiety about speaking, but they seldom cure the disability completely. Children with mild disfluencies and adults who stutter slightly with few associated anxieties can often be helped without too much difficulty, but full-blown, severe stuttering in adults poses real problems for the therapist and the patient.

People have been trying to find the cause of stuttering and the remedy for more than two thousand years, but until recently they didn't have much success. During the heyday of the Greek and Roman empires, attention focused on stutterers' speech machinery, particularly the tongue, and this approach persisted until the last half of the nineteenth century. It was widely assumed that stuttering was caused by a physical disability, but at the same time efforts were made to divert the stutterer's attention away from his speech by various devices.

By the end of the nineteenth century, the influence of Freud led clinicians to try to treat the alleged psychological abnormalities that they supposed were the cause of stuttering. During the present century, people who stutter have been subjected to a barrage of different treatments, among them breath control, elocution, relaxation, distraction, sound, pills, hypnosis, ventriloquism, conditioning, and speech training.

Since the 1930s the trend has been to treat the stutterer as a whole person, modifying his attitudes as well as his speech; modern conditioning techniques, too, have helped to deal with the problems. The current trend is to use the particular combination of techniques that seems best suited to an individual. Scientists are still looking for an organic cause that will respond to medication.

With all these treatments available to stutterers, you'd think that there would be something to help everybody. Unfortunately this is not quite the case. Treatments not only take a long time but can also be expensive and often make great demands on the patient's emotional stamina. Not all people are able to receive or persist with treatment. There is also still a tendency for those who become fluent in the clinic to relapse into disfluency in the outside world. Recent sophisticated approaches are reducing the number of relapses, but regression into disfluency is still common – and frustrating for both the therapist and the patient. Even after fifty-five years of therapy I still relapse when I am tired, careless, or anxious.

Historically, the treatment of stutters has been empirical, and it still is to a large extent; if a treatment worked it was used, even though the underlying reasons were not fully understood. Unfortunately, many treatments help only for a short time.

Although many of the early treatments look absurd today, the therapists of the past were doing their best to deal with a malady they did not understand. A great deal more is now known, although we still cannot fit together all the pieces in the jigsaw. Some are missing and others don't fit very well; but the outlines of the picture are gradually beginning to emerge. There is every reason to believe that stuttering will yield to modern science.

What follows describes the early gropings for solutions during the Dark Ages of speech therapy together with the methods used in the transition period before the 1930s, when many theories were tested, and most were found to be wrong. The emergence of modern therapy with its twin thrusts of treating the whole person and conditioning him to speak more fluently are then outlined. The attempt is made to describe a complex subject as simply as possible. If at times my descriptions stray from the solid path of fact and flounder in the mud of conjecture, I am in good company.

The Dark Ages of speech therapy

For centuries, treating stuttering has been a bonanza for quacks. Few treatments are likely to be lethal except for some of the more ill-advised surgical procedures, so a charlatan whose treatment fails isn't likely to be sued. He can always say the patient didn't co-operate or persevere with the treatment.

As early as the fifth century BC, the famous physician Hippocrates (460–400 BC) concluded that stuttering was caused by a dry tongue and prescribed substances to blister the tongue and remove the black bile responsible for the disfluency. Many stutterers have dry mouths because they are frequently anxious about speaking, and Hippocrates confused cause with effect.

A century later the Greek philosopher Aristotle (384–322 BC) agreed that stuttering (which he called 'ischnophonoi') had something to do with the tongue. He also felt that coldness impeded the speech, but had the wisdom not to prescribe treatments.

While Aristotle was acting as mentor to Alexander the Great in Macedonia, the great orator Demosthenes was making a great deal of trouble in Athens with his caustic tongue, stirring up opposition to Alexander's father, Philip of Macedon. Demosthenes seems to have been remarkably testy and articulate. Nevertheless historians tell us that he suffered from a speech defect, allegedly stuttering, and overcame his problem by placing pebbles under his tongue and shouting above the thunder of the waves pounding the coast of Greece. Modern therapists feel that he distracted his attention away from his speech, but the roaring waves may have masked his voice and made him more fluent. Speaking loudly helps some people with their stuttering for a short period, so his approach was triple-barrelled.

During the first century BC, the philosopher Celsus tried to treat stuttering as a physician and as a surgeon. His prescriptions were bad enough. He advised people plagued by stuttering to carry out breathing exercises, wash the head in cold water, eat horseradish, and vomit, which sounds socially messy. His surgical techniques at a time when anaesthesia and aseptic procedures were regarded as unnecessary sound horrendous. Following the guidelines of a doctor called Aetius, he lifted the tongue, stretched the membrane on the underside with a hook, and carefully cut the membrane all the way through with a sharp knife. The mouth was then rinsed with a mixture of vinegar and water, called *'posca'*, followed by powdered frankincense and manna, a solidified honeydew.

Some patients had their speech restored, but there was often profuse bleeding. An alternative was to perforate the membrane with a needle, draw a thread through the hole, and tie it into a knot. The thread was gradually tightened and slowly amputated the membrane. The wound was 'consumed' by Egyptian ointment and drying powders to prevent the membrane from forming again. As one commentator later wrote, 'this is a most agreeable method.' One wonders for whom.[1]

Persuasion and faith were also used to treat stuttering. A Greek prince named Batthus, who apparently stuttered very badly, consulted the famous Oracle at Delphi about what he should do to cure his handicap. The Oracle advised him to go abroad and never return, one of the earliest examples of brushing an intractable complaint under the medical carpet. Batthus gathered together an army and sailed to North Africa where he managed to control his stuttering enough to vanquish his enemies and become governor of Cyrene. Many stutterers find that a change of environment and success in life help their speech for a while. The Delphic Oracle was not all that far out of line.

Incidentally, Batthus (sometimes called Batarus) tended to repeat the first syllable of each word and lent his name to the speech defect known in medieval times as *'batarismus.'*[2]

During the Middle Ages, physicians' attention still focused on the tongue in the tradition of Hippocrates and Aristotle. Some unfortunates with stutters had their tongues burned to encourage fluency, and no doubt they made every effort to overcome their problem and avoid the treatment.

About this time doctors had another look at the idea that dryness of the body, particularly of the tongue, caused stuttering. Strange prescriptions were offered to stutterers, such as gargling with woman's milk or rinsing the mouth with an infusion of boiled water-lily leaves. Dampening the tongue with water mallow, oil of almonds, water lily, and saffron was also thought to help stutterers with their speech.[3]

In 1584 Hieronymous Mercurialis, a famous physician who based his work on Galen's idea that people's behaviour and

health were controlled by the four bodily humours (blood –
the sanguine; phlegm – the phlegmatic; bile – the choleric;
and water – the melancholic), wrote what was probably the
first complete overview of stuttering in a book on childhood
diseases. He recommended that a person with a stutter remain in warm, dry conditions, avoid outbreaks of anger, and
refrain from making love, drinking wine, and eating pastry,
nuts, or fish. Poultices were prescribed, and the patients were
told to speak loudly and forcefully, maintain bowel activity,
and engage in vigorous physical exercise. He advocated a
strenuous and boring life. I wonder how many of his patients
persisted with the treatment.[4]

Mercurialis's treatment was fairly benign. Much later, in
the middle of the nineteenth century, treatment of stutterers
was more drastic. In 1841, the famous Prussian surgeon, Dr
Dieffenbach, developed a surgical procedure to cure stuttering that was sheer butchery. Like Hippocrates and Celsus he
thought that the source of the trouble was the tongue, so he
cut large wedges from the tongues of many patients with stutters. His procedure was copied in both Europe and the
United States at a time before effective anaesthetics and
sterile procedures were widely used. Several patients died in
agony. The pain and distress of the victims do not bear thinking about, and the treatment is a dark blot on the history of
speech therapy.[5]

During the nineteenth century several surgical treatments
of the tongue, the tonsils, and the palate were used in attempts to relieve speech disorders. Cutting the tongue's
frenulum, which connects the underside of the tongue to the
floor of the mouth, was thought to be beneficial by allowing
more freedom of movement. Luchsinger and Arnold felt that
this surgery had as much value as clipping someone's toe-
nails to cure a walking disorder.[6]

I suspect that I was indirectly the victim of one of these
misguided procedures in the early 1930s when tonsillectomies
were almost a ritual for young boys aged about ten, like a second circumcision. The surgeons used the operation to maintain their cash flows. I'd had a sore throat for a while, and an
elderly surgeon, who wore a bow-tie, tails, and spats, decided
to whip out my tonsils, adding that it would 'probably cure

his stutter.' He was right. The ham-fisted fellow broke my jaw, and since I couldn't speak in more than a mumble, for a while I had no trouble with stuttering whatsoever.

Some wily entrepreneurs have lined their pockets by selling strange devices for stutterers to wear in their mouths while speaking. I never used these contraptions but saw one in London, England, that looked like a ferocious rat trap, all plates and springs. Even respected physicians have recommended gadgets like a golden fork attached to the teeth to exercise and strengthen the tongue.[7]

Anybody interested in the more macabre side of medicine should read Murray Katz's 1977 'Survey of patented anti-stuttering devices.'[8] The technical drawings of the devices are reminiscent of designs for the furnishing of medieval torture chambers, complete with enough gags, spikes, levers, clamps, nutcrackers, shafts, springs, grids, belts, and tubes to scare anybody into fluency. Most of these toys were registered in the first half of this century. Some kept the air passages open (to yell for help?), some prevented the stutterer from clenching his teeth, others exercised or immobilized the tongue muscles, and a few co-ordinated breathing and speaking. One little beauty consisted of a spiked reed attached to the roof of the mouth. When the stutterer breathed out it whistled and helped him to maintain his airflow. If he moved his tongue incorrectly, the spike pricked the offending member, goading the speaker along the paths of articulacy. The responses of stutterers to these devices is not recorded. My response is quite definite. Sheer terror!

A physician once advised me to clamp the stem of an unlit pipe between my teeth when I spoke to stabilize my lips. My jaws ached most of the time, and it made me sound like a stuttering ventriloquist. One lady, a Madame Leigh, persuaded the French government to pay her several hundred thousand francs for her secret cure for stuttering, which consisted of a pad of cotton wool beneath the tongue. It may have reduced some of the speech tremors and was far better than some of the junk that experts have told stutterers to stick in their mouths.

People afflicted by stuttering have suffered a great deal at the hands of physicians with little knowledge about stuttering who nevertheless administered drugs or therapy based on reports half remembered from their student days. Over a period of forty years, well-meaning practitioners have prescribed for me tranquillizers, stimulants, vitamins, pills to improve muscular co-ordination, purgatives (!), exercises, diets, learning French, and illicit love. Fortunately I knew enough about my speech not to comply with most of them, although the last one attracted my interest. It would not have surprised me in the least to have been offered leeches to relieve my system of surplus blood to take the pressure off my stuttering. People who stutter should look askance at any prescription that is not based on a thorough clinical assessment by a qualified speech pathologist. The Dark Ages of speech therapy ended all too recently.

A matter of faith

Faith is such a rare and precious commodity that it cannot be consigned to the rag-bag of unsuccessful stuttering remedies and pushed away out of sight. Any stutterer entering intensive therapy must have faith in himself, the therapist, and the treatment or he should stay at home and make room for a patient with better motivation. The faith healers and those practitioners outside the medical profession who use unorthodox suggestion and vibration techniques sometimes have remarkable results with sick people, particularly those whose conditions are complicated by emotional problems. A person with a stutter is a prime target for treatment by these methods.

One stuttering friend paid large sums of money to a well-known faith healer in Europe who assured him that the donations would be used for charitable purposes. This practitioner clearly hadn't taken a vow of poverty; after all, charity begins at home. In spite of my doubts, my friend's speech improved tremendously for the two years I knew him.

The only faith healer I ever met was staying at a small, unheated hotel in an isolated part of northern Europe in the middle of winter. We were drawn together more by a mutual need of body heat than by any intellectual affinity. He was a great man for vibrations and laying on of hands and insisted on trying them out on me after dinner one night. I suspect that his laying on of hands was an excuse to warm his finger tips, but he came up with the diagnosis that my problem lay in a bit of bone on my frontispiece called the sternum. He told me that if I had faith and rubbed the bone every night with a mixture of vinegar and honey, my stuttering would disappear. He didn't charge me a fee, which surprised me, because he was in the area to use his vibes to find hidden gold in a peat bog. I'm afraid I didn't test his method.

In spite of the encounter with my vibrating friend, it is possible that any therapy that results in a marked change in a person's attitude toward himself, his goals and philosophy, his speech, and the people around him could affect his fluency considerably. Anything that relieves some of his anxiety about speaking is sure to be beneficial. Some unorthodox practitioners hit the right spot by accident, others do it by building up real faith.

Stand and deliver: elocution

Prior to World War II, when speech therapists were still groping in the dark, a large number of people set up businesses in Britain as elocutionists to teach dramatic delivery, remove unfashionable accents, and overcome stuttering. The practitioners were usually retired actors and actresses (with names like James Mayhew, Esquire, and Madame Lear) who believed sincerely that any speech defect could be cured by breathing and enunciating correctly and by projecting the voice in the correct manner. They had been on the stage long before amplifiers, woofers, and tweeters were used, and were very keen on *projection*, because they had to be heard up in the *gods*, the upper, upper circle. As one good lady with a queen-sized operatic bust said, 'A parrot can speak, my dear, but he cannot PROJECT.' The windows rattled.

I passed through several elocutionists' hands, including those of one dragon lady who whomped our heads with her conductor's baton whenever we mangled our words. The finest of all was a blue-eyed, jolly, Falstaffian actor with pendulous jowls, long, white, silky hair, and a booming voice. His name was Ryder Boyes, and I met him when I was twelve years of age. He had been on the stage with Sir Henry Irving – he proudly showed me the silver-headed cane given to him by the great man – and his rooms were full of theatrical memorabilia and signed photographs of Victorian and Edwardian thespians. He loved language, and even more he loved people.

For months he taught me how to 'breathe from the belly,' 'stand up and deliver,' and 'project,' until one day he asked me to his home for tea and a man-to-man talk. He said it was clear that he couldn't cure my stutter, so he would teach me how to live with it. For one hour every week for a year he taught me love of life, love of people, and love of words, supported by appropriate quotations from Shakespeare. He insisted that I should value myself and face the world with 'the bright blade of honour, courage, and determination.' It was hard for a small boy with a stutter to wield a bright blade when most of his teachers called him a fool in spite of his good grades, but old Ryder Boyes's jowls would quiver and his voice boom with anger whenever he heard my resolution falter. For the sum of one guinea a week I received Darjeeling tea (with no milk), fruity Dundee cake, and the best counselling in the world. My speech steadily improved for several years. Ryder Boyes – across the years I salute you!

The trouble with elocution was that it focused a stutterer's attention on his speech and, because the teachers were largely theatrical artists, rewarded perfection and performance. Most of the teachers had little platforms for you to stand on and *deliver*, while the other sufferers giggled at your inarticulacy. The classes tended to recreate the social pressures that may have precipitated the stuttering in the first place.

Nevertheless, some of these elocutionists had success. Charles Van Riper describes one woman who helped stutterers by drilling them in mental arithmetic.[9] The stutterers were mostly poor, deprived children with low school grades and even lower morale. The elocutionist ignored their stuttering and gave the children love, faith, and patience, as well as a facility with mental arithmetic that amazed the other children, the teachers, and the parents. The speech of some of the children improved. Like Ryder Boyes, she increased their self-confidence and self-regard.

The limp rag in a steel world: relaxation

When a stutterer speaks he often appears to be nervous, tense and agitated. For centuries it was thought that the agitation caused the stutter, when in fact the reverse seems to be true. During the nineteenth century the therapist Sandow taught stutterers how to relax when they spoke, and many found that their fluency greatly improved, although this improvement was only temporary.[10] Since anxiety and struggling to speak often disappear when a patient is deeply relaxed, this type of therapy works fairly well until the stutterer is thrust into competitive society where relaxation is difficult or even impossible. As Van Riper said, it is hard to be a limp rag in a steel world. Anxiety and struggles of one kind or another are just parts of normal life.

Relaxation therapy reached a peak of popularity during the 1930s, and for a short time I participated in a class in northern Britain. We assembled in a gymnasium smelling strongly of sweaty gymnasts and did relaxation exercises on dusty mats that made us sneeze. The teacher, a well-endowed young woman, taught us to think peaceful thoughts and achieve tranquillity by closing our eyes, breathing deeply, and exhaling slowly with a faint hissing sound. When relaxed we were urged to speak on any topic that came to our minds.

My problem was that the young teacher was so attractive that, like all the other young men in her class, I could not resist peeking at her magnificent endowments through my eyelashes. My thoughts were not particularly peaceful and my feelings were far from tranquil, so relaxation was out of the question.

On the few occasions when I managed to relax completely, I just fell asleep on the floor and had lurid dreams. Even when I managed to control my adolescent urges, relax, stay awake, and speak all at the same time, I still stumbled and bumbled over my words. Some of the older members of the class who stuttered less severely had some luck and became quite fluent in the clinic.

Relaxation therapy is still widely used. From my own experience it was most valuable as a part of a wider therapeutic approach involving complete speech rehabilitation. During such therapy the patients can become very tense, and relaxation helps to increase the effectiveness of the other therapies.

Many therapists look on relaxation techniques with scepticism, but anything that makes people relax a little without using drugs in the headlong dash of modern living has a place.

Distraction

Distractive methods direct the attention of the stutterer away from his speech. Many have been successful in the clinics, but there has been much less success in the conditions of everyday life. Distraction techniques include rhythmics, some forms of speech training, devices such as corks between the teeth or pads beneath the tongue, chewing, shrugging, whistling, counting, ventriloquism, and smoking a pipe. Delayed auditory feedback and use of speech maskers have also been regarded as distractions, but that is an over-simplification.

I first met distraction therapy in 1936. I had fallen in the school workshop and struck my head on the sharp edge of a large metal vise, neatly splitting my scalp and producing spectacular pools of gore. I was rushed to the doctor bleeding all over the teacher's Austin Seven, and endured the shaving of a freeway across my head, followed by the painful attachment of six metal clips like silvery hockey pucks along the incision. While he worked, the doctor chatted about my speech to take my mind off the pain.

When I returned for treatment a few days later he made me tap my foot and speak at the same time, with little success. On the next visit he had me speaking while I crawled all over his Persian carpet on all fours. This worked quite well, but, like any small boy, I couldn't help going off into fits of giggles at the thought of going back to school and asking questions on my hands and knees.

This treatment may sound like the height of medical absurdity, but the doctor had done his homework. I found out years later that at about that time a scientist called Geniesse[11] had discovered that timing stutterers' speech with their movements while they crawled around on all fours significantly increased their fluency. The physician was not as daft as I thought he was. The technique poses obvious social hazards, and if I were to go to a restaurant and order my meal on all fours the *maître d'hotel* could be forgiven for either calling the police or offering me a doggy-bag.

A well-meaning school teacher introduced me to an innovative therapy that he claimed would distract my attention from my speech, improve my breathing, and help my fluency. He was the Officers' Training Corps bandmaster and was short of buglers. What could be more sensible than to recruit me into the discordant brass and show me how to blow that strident and unlovely instrument, the bugle? I spent a week making wet, hissing noises down the coiled tube, with an apoplectic face and the imprint of the circular mouthpiece on my swollen lips. My breathing was a total disaster. I never did get the hang of blowing and speaking at the same time, so it didn't help the stutter at all. I was dismissed in disgrace from the wind section, and I have a feeling that if the band had needed a big bass drum thumper, the bass drum would have been prescribed as speech therapy.

One of the distractions that frequently improves fluency is intense fear. During World War II there were many instances of stutterers becoming fluent in moments of intense crisis. Some soldiers and air crew found that they spoke quite normally in action and stuttered badly when at home on leave. This appears to be illogical when fear is so closely associated with the roots of stuttering, but Bloodstein[12] makes the point that it is not just anxiety that precipitates stuttering, but anxiety about stuttering.

Rhythmics have played a major role in distractive stuttering therapy for more than a century. As early as 1837, Serre d'Alais used an instrument called an isochrome, which produced a rhythmic beat for the stutterer to follow when he spoke.[13] The well-known and sometimes infamous stuttering schools leaned heavily on rhythmics because they were fairly sure to get good short-term responses from most of the patients in the clinical situation. The stuttering would completely disappear while the patients spoke to a rhythm as they marched, swung their arms, tapped their feet and fingers, timed their speech syllables with metronomes, nodded their heads, and danced. I was told to march and swing my arms when I spoke, but this didn't work too well at formal dinner parties.

I learned to use my pulse as a metronome and measure my rate of speaking at the same time. My pulse rate was about seventy beats a minute, so it helped to keep my rate of speaking below 80 words a minute, which is my most controllable rate. When I speak faster than 120 words a minute my speech falls apart. The trouble was that everybody thought I was listening to my pulse in case I had a heart attack. The pulse monitor didn't work under pressure, but I still use it occasionally to time my speaking rate.

A portable rhythmic device, developed by Meyer and Mair in 1963,[14] looked like a hearing aid and delivered a rhythmic beat that enabled stutterers to time their speech without embarrassment. The patients slowly became less dependent on the device as their speech improved, but unfortunately they tended to relapse.

The effectiveness of the rhythmic beat depends upon its rate. About ninety beats per minute seems to be the best rate. Faster or more irregular beats are less effective.[15] Some feel that improvement in fluency from rhythmic therapy may not be caused merely by distraction. The rhythm reduces the rate of speaking to levels stutterers can manage, as with my heartbeat. There is also some evidence that rhythm itself, quite apart from its distraction and control of speech rate, can modify the speech by making the time of the speech sounds more predictable. Rhythmic therapy may be much more than distraction and is still used in some schools of stuttering.

Rhythmics and other tricks taught by the earlier therapists (tricks like articulating a glottal stop before a hard word) have the drawback that they are inclined to leave a legacy of undesirable tics and mannerisms. Any therapy that uses speech tricks, starters, or physical movements can have undesirable residual effects. I still tend to twitch my hand and leg when I stutter, a throwback to rhythmic therapy of thirty years ago when I was taught to tap my foot and hand to get through a block. One man was taught to clench his right hand when he stuttered 'to stimulate the left side of the brain' where right-handed people have their speech and language centre. He did this so well that he developed huge muscles on his right arm in contrast to his skinny left.

Phonation therapy (or resonance therapy) was used in some of the large hospitals in Britain during the 1930s and 1940s. In some ways this therapy was simply speech training, because it taught control of air flow and the vocal chords; but it also contained a large element of distraction.

Following World War II my speech was at a low ebb. I was not so bad as some stutterers whom the stresses of war had reduced to total mutes, but my ability to communicate was so limited that the Armed Forces sponsored my treatment at a large London hospital. The therapist was a man in his late fifties with a distinctly military, no-nonsense air. Treatment was on a one-to-one basis with no opportunity to compare notes with other patients. The therapist was a bully, and we didn't get on at all well. He started the therapy with a finger-wagging homily about how all his patients had recovered, so I had better maintain his record, and continued with the warning that I would become a social outcast, etc., etc., unless I stopped stuttering. It was all a bit threatening and discouraging.

The therapy had none of today's psychological frills. You established a fundamental, low-frequency, resonant tone by uttering the prolonged sound 'er,' and checking with your fingertips to see that your larynx was vibrating. You maintained this basic monotone, thereby keeping up the airflow, and superimposed your words. I tried this for a week with little success, because my speech was so bad that I blocked on the 'er' and couldn't resonate most of the time. When I could resonate, the words I tried to superimpose just wouldn't come out. The therapist became impatient and angry, and I protested (with a stutter) that asking me to say 'er' and superimpose my words on the sound was like telling a short-sighted person without glasses to read small-print instructions on how to improve his sight.

This miserable business went on for six months and my speech became worse and worse. I learned to say the 'er' and resonate, but nothing else, and my voice fixed on the monotone. The 'er' became a vocalized block that I couldn't go beyond. When I met people, instead of saying, 'Hello', I just said 'Er,' which limited further conversation, and I began to associate therapy and speaking with increased frustration and anger. The authoritarian therapist may have helped some patients, but for me the treatment was a disaster. It took me three years to recover from the conditioned 'er'

block. The therapist retired before my treatment was co_
pleted, so he kept his score of 100 per cent success.

Very few therapists I met were bullies. Most were firm and
demanding, but in a positive way. The only other bullies I
met were young male trainees who, feeling their power over
the patients, created superior-subordinate relationships. The
patients soon let these young men know their displeasure. It
was all part of the trainees' learning process. A rapport between patient and therapist is vital.

The clinician was not necessarily lying when he said that all
his resonating patients recovered. They may have done so in
the clinic, but it is doubtful that many maintained their fluency in the workplace and under social pressures.

This therapy, like many others, used one approach for all
patients and did not take into account the different needs of
individuals. My martinet created an atmosphere of anxiety,
hostility, and guilt that modern therapists avoid at all costs,
because these emotions are cues to stutter.

There are many other methods of distraction. The trouble
with all of them is that the patient is delighted when he
becomes fluent for a while and is shattered with disappointment when he later plunges back into disfluency. One man
made me say tongue-twisters before every therapy session to
distract me, saying that if I could focus on the difficult words
the ordinary words would be easy. I could say 'Peggy Bab-
cock' and 'Black Bug's Blood' five times quickly without
hesitation, but saying 'Good morning' still defeated me.
Distraction involves avoiding facing up to the stuttering
squarely. It is a mere escape hatch. Like anybody else with a
handicap, a person with a severe stutter cannot afford to run
away from his problem.

Auditory feedback

Auditory feedback refers to the feedback of the sounds of
speech to a person's ear. Delayed auditory feedback (DAF)
tends to disrupt the speech, and when sound is used to prevent a stutterer from hearing his own speech his fluency often
increases. Both of these facts have been used to treat stuttering.

The therapeutic use of DAF arose from research on effects of conditioning stutterers using reward and punishment. The stutterer was exposed to continuous delayed (0.2 second) auditory feedback of his speech. When he was relieved from the disruptive, delayed feedback for ten seconds each time he blocked, he responded by speaking in a slow, prolonged, and more fluent manner, so DAF was used to develop slow, prolonged speech. The delayed sound was slowly reduced and normal speech rates gradually restored. There seemed to be some carry-over of the improved speech from the clinic to ordinary life.[16]

It is not clear whether DAF is effective simply because it distracts the stutterer from his speech, but even if it is a distraction the carry-over seems to be better than with rhythmic methods and gadgets in the mouth.

My attention was first drawn to the masking technique in 1957 by Professor E.T. Jones, a physicist who played a major role as a scientific boffin during World War II. At his suggestion I visited a laboratory in northwestern England to test a prototype of a masking instrument consisting of a heavy tape recorder delivering loud continuous white sound (mixed frequencies) to a pair of large earphones. My speech at that time was very disfluent, but the continuous noise at a level of about 100 decibels enabled me to read aloud fluently in the clinic. Unfortunately, the benefit faded when I tried the instrument at home. I could still read aloud and recite, but couldn't combine my thoughts and speech to convey information, because the stuttering cues in the words still overrode the effects of the sound. The noise gave me a headache and, instead of getting used to it, I became irritated by it. Continuous white sound is now known to be less effective in increasing fluency than low frequency (500 Hz) sound delivered only when the stutterer speaks.

In 1976 the masking technique was refined by Ann Dewar and her colleagues at Edinburgh University, Scotland,[17] but I didn't consider testing it because I was responding well to other speech therapy, although I still had great difficulty using the telephone and speaking to audiences of more than a few people.

I instinctively distrust gadgets, particularly those used in

speech therapy, but when I heard that Ann Dewar's Edin-
burgh Masker was being manufactured by Findlay, Irvine
Ltd., at Penicuik, Scotland, and distributed in Canada by
Cantechs Ltd., of St John, New Brunswick, and in the
United States by the Foundation for Fluency, Inc., of
Chicago, Illinois, I decided to test the instrument for a
month.

The Edinburgh Masker consists of a neat little electronic
sound-producer or buzzer about the size of a packet of
cigarettes, a throat microphone, a small junction box, and
ear-pieces. The sound producer makes a low-pitched hum, of
about 500 Hz, which is modified by the pitch of the speaker's
voice and has a noise level of about ninety decibels. When a
person speaks, the throat microphone turns the buzzer on
and turns it off again when he stops, with a small lag to allow
for normal pauses in speech. The buzzer unit has a manual
switch that can override the throat microphone when necessary. Some ear-pieces are of the stethoscope type, but more
comfortable skeletal ear-moulds are available. The sound is
conveyed from the buzzer to the ear-pieces by small tubes
made of clear plastic, and the conventional throat microphone is attached to a point just below the Adam's apple by a
fabric tape. The microphone gets uncomfortable on hot days,
but it can be replaced by a smaller throat microphone attached by two-way sticky pads to the throat. If a person is
wearing a collar and tie or a turtle-neck sweater, the apparatus is no more obstrusive than a hearing-aid. (With an
open-neck shirt, however, it looks as though the wearer has
had a tracheotomy.)

The noise level is fairly high, and there was the possibility
that the masker would damage a user's hearing. Taking into
account the average number of hours the stutterers wore the
masker (3.3 hours per day) and the average period they spoke
(about 7.5 minutes per hour) Ann Dewar found that the
sound exposure was within the official limits for workers.
Careful monitoring of seventeen patients' hearing for up to
three years failed to detect any reduction in hearing acuity at
any sound frequency.[18]

The Edinburgh University team found that a lawyer and a
pharmacist spoke very little (2.8 to 3.2 minutes each hour)

during an ordinary working day, a university lecturer spoke much more (9.3 minutes each hour), while a retail salesman, a physiotherapist, and an interior decorator all spoke a great deal (11.6 to 13.4 minutes each hour). Nobody spoke much more than three hours each day, so the exposure to the noise was relatively short.[19]

Sixty-seven users of the masker were tested in Britain over a two-year period; 42 per cent received great benefit, 40 per cent considerable benefit, and 18 per cent slight benefit. Some objected to the appearance of the instrument, and others didn't like the noise. However, most thought that the benefits outweighed the disadvantages. About 70 per cent of the patients found that the instrument remained effective for a year at least; others found that the benefit declined. Five patients became fully fluent and discarded the instrument.[20]

The Edinburgh Masker's effects surprised me. I expected the blanking out of my speech by the sound to produce fluency for a while; but since I regarded it as a mere distraction and my stutter is an intractable type, I didn't expect much more. I had used distractive techniques before and their effects soon faded.

I tested the masker in stores and on the telephone, and there were a few failures, some the result of minor malfunctions of the instrument and others of my own attitude. I tried, without realizing it, to hear my own voice above the noise, in a desperate attempt to get feedback. When I succeeded, I stuttered. I tended to use the override too much, relying on the continuous noise rather than larynx-activated noise, but I stopped this when I learned to trust the throat microphone.

I had some early difficulties controlling the loudness of my speech and varying my voice's pitch. I tended to speak in a loud monotone like some deaf people, but I mastered these problems in two days. The noise was irritating at first, but I soon became used to it.

Since my family tells me that I talk too much even with my stuttering, I had to curb the urge to monopolize the conversation. I couldn't hear interruptions when I spoke, and it didn't give people a chance to chip in. I learned to watch people as I spoke and to let them have their say. The instrument worked best for me if I spoke in the slow, prolonged manner I had been taught by the excellent speech therapists at the Royal Ottawa Hospital. Without the masker I had to keep an iron control on my speech to use the techniques, but with the instrument it was much easier, and I could relax a little. There was less tension and less need to focus my attention on the approach to every sentence. Somebody who knew me said, 'What's happened to your speech?' and hadn't noticed the ear-moulds and throat microphone. I was fairly fluent apart from normal disfluency and fumbling for the right word.

It appears that the masker, quite apart from its distraction, removes the effect of most of my stuttering cues. I can read aloud, and words beginning with 'm,' 'p,' 'b,' and 't' no longer cause my stomach to tense as I prepare to cope. I don't anticipate a struggle. It helps my automatic speech and defuses most of my anxiety about stuttering.

Some cues still make me block even with a masker. If I visualize my name in writing, I have to make a great effort to keep control by using prolonged speech even though I cannot hear myself, but when I say my name automatically without seeing the words I am fluent.

My controllable rate of speaking has risen to 140 words a minute, which is easier on the listener. I was also startled to find that, after using the masker for several hours, I was much more fluent for a day or more afterwards, even when I did not use the device.

The machine isn't foolproof, and you don't just switch it on and speak. The user has to learn to stop trying to hear himself, and avoid visual images of his cues to block.

So far, so good. I intend to test the masker in more challenging situations – in committee meetings, on radio and television, and when speaking in public. The benefit may fade, but the masker makes me much more fluent on the telephone, which was always my worst cue to stutter, so I am cautiously optimistic. I shall also maintain the speech techniques I learned earlier.

Some therapists vehemently oppose the use of portable masking devices, and Sheehan[21] pointed out that they lend themselves to quackery. The masker does not help some people, and with others the benefit sometimes fades. The possibility that the masking sound may act merely as a distraction or avoidance raises the hackles of some therapists, and the haphazard, unguided use of the masker is not recommended. I just describe how it works for me.

Why the masker helps I don't know. It is not undoing previous therapy, or changing my attitudes. I have a verbal limp, and the masker helps me, like a walking-stick rather than a crutch, over the rough ground. If the masker continues to work I shall be delighted, and if the effect fades I shall be philosophical. To deny older stutterers who have been through the therapeutic mill a little help on the grounds of principle seems a little dogmatic.

Some younger stutterers find that a masking device helps them to lead normal lives, and good luck to them so long as they realize that they may need treatment for behavioural and attitudinal problems. If wearing a funny nose and plastic vampire teeth helps them to communicate and keeps them happy, I'd still say good luck.

The use of the masker, without previous professional assessment, by children, adolescents, and young adults is ill-advised. It's rather like giving a walking-stick to someone with an untreated paralysed leg. People with severe stutters often need rehabilitative therapy quite apart from modification of the speech.

The machine could be improved. There are still minor bugs such as kinked tubes, faulty cables, and erratic microphone contact, and ways of using it need tailoring to the individual. Nevertheless there are grounds for cautious optimism.

Some successful users report a complete change in their lives and attitudes, but I have not found this to be the case. It is easier to speak to people, interview editors, talk on the telephone, and order meals, but I used to do all these things before, stutter or no stutter. The masker just makes life easier and reduces anxieties about speaking.

Magic pills

At one time I kept a collection of pills that various physicians had prescribed for my stuttering over a period of ten years.

Many of the bottles remained unopened. All were kept in a locked cupboard because some were remarkably potent. There were enough tiny phenobarbitone tablets to put a small village to sleep. Beside them on the shelf were two brown bottles labelled 'Serenase' and 'Stematil.' Serapasil (or reserpine) kept company with the stimulant Benzedrine, and a small, dark, sinister bottle containing sodium amytal had a paper tag on which I had written 'Not Bloody Likely!' There were some little yellow pills that were supposed to improve a spastic's co-ordination (they made me sick after my one and only dose), vitamins B and C, and several unopened bottles of the tranquillizers chlorpromazine and Meprobamate. I never spent money on these pills because the physicians were a little casual about drugs and gave me pills off their sample shelves like candies. After a few unfortunate experiences I became cautious, and eventually the pills were flushed down the lavatorial bend.

The physicians who provided the drugs meant well, but they had no expertise in speech pathology. Many worked on the vague premise that relaxing a stutterer would cure his speech. Some doctors also had the idea that, since people who stutter severely sometimes look depressed (who wouldn't if they couldn't speak?) they just need a good belt of Benzedrine to tune up their systems.

About that time researchers were testing drugs on stutterers, and the physician who prescribed the Serpasil (reserpine), chlorpromazine, and Meprobamate had probably kept up with the scientific literature. These drugs reduce anxiety and tension in stutterers and have been beneficial as part of other therapy. Nevertheless, the results from the experiments were conflicting, and there is no unquestionable evidence that the drugs alleviate stuttering.[22]

While drugs such as tranquillizers can be useful in speech therapy and the treatment of other disorders, whether they are used depends upon the balance between the adverse side effects and the potential benefits. Some drugs have slight effects while others are potent, selective toxins.

Serpasil (or reserpine) has been widely used to treat high blood pressure and to sedate tense stutterers. This drug is now suspected of being associated with breast cancer and can have a wide range of side effects, including nausea, depression, sleeplessness, nightmares, drowsiness, and dizziness. Many other drugs react with reserpine in a harmful manner.

Meprobamate releases tensions, but can result in hives, clumsiness, drowsiness, blurred vision, diarrhoea, headaches, tiredness, and nausea and is not prescribed for pregnant women. It can slow the speech, suggesting some effect on the speech or language centres, and reacts with such drugs as antihistamines, narcotics, and barbiturates. Use of chlorpromazine, one of the phenothiazines, can cause muscle spasms, restlessness, tics, trembling, and sometimes fainting. The side effects vary from person to person, but many people adjust to these medicines after a short time.[23]

Other types of medication besides tranquillizers have been used to help stutterers. Heavy doses of vitamins B and C apparently benefit some people who stutter, but information on the duration of the improvement is hard to find. A physician prescribed for me large quantities of vitamin B-complex capsules, which resulted in a feeling of well-being but had no effect on my speech. The capsules are not, of course, as potent or effective as the massive vitamin injections given to some stutterers. It is difficult to see how vitamins can deal with the numerous factors that mediate a stutter.

So far nobody has invented the magic pill that will make stutterers completely fluent, and it isn't likely that anyone will do so, unless the predisposition to stutter is found to have an organic, neurological origin in some abnormality in the brain's speech centres. Neurological abnormality could possibly be treated by hormones or biochemicals that modify neurotransmitters. Even if this were possible it may not help adults with their Pandora's boxes of haunting anxieties about speech opened in childhood by the key of society's demands.

It is now clear that simple relaxation, by chemical or other means, will not resolve many stutterers' problems outside the clinic, and stimulants aren't likely to help, either; the stutter itself stimulates most people who stutter more than they wish. Perhaps, as the new schools of behavioural biology and physiology unravel the biochemical mysteries of our emotions and behaviour, they will shed light on the biochemical processes of anxiety-conditioned disabilities like stuttering and show us how to deal with them.

The power of suggestion

Surely somebody can persuade stutterers that there's no need to be anxious about the bats in their vocal belfries, and that they should stop all the fuss and bother of avoiding stuttering and get on with the business of automatic, fluent, controlled speaking. I trained a budgerigar under a black cloth to say 'Douglas (my brother), silly boy,' so it shouldn't be too hard to put me in a dark room and persuade me to mimic fluent speech.

A few people may have been made fluent by hypnosis. Unfortunately, the effect doesn't usually persist beyond the hypnotic trance, and the speech can relapse to a worse state than before. It is not as though the practitioners of hypnosis are trying to correct organic disorders like blindness or deafness, because a stutterer shows by his spells of fluency that he has all the necessary articulatory equipment. It should be possible to persuade him to use it. Sad to say, hypnosis doesn't usually work.

Suggestion plays a hidden role in most modern speech therapy. When the therapy includes psychotherapy and counselling, a skilled clinician will guide a stutterer to persuade himself to adopt certain attitudes and to speak in certain ways. One patient went to a qualified practitioner with a view to using hypnotic suggestion to reduce his hang-ups about speaking. After a few months of discussion, the patient asked when the hypnosis would start. The doctor replied that it had nearly finished, because the patient had used suggestion on himself and was greatly improved.

Every therapist uses non-hypnotic suggestion in speech classes, because it takes a great deal of gentle persuasion to get the stutterer to carry out projects like stopping strangers on the street to ask the way to the bus station or post office while repeating sounds deliberately. The nervous patient is likely to hide in a coffee shop. The therapist cannot bludgeon the stutterer into carrying out the painful tasks. She must make him feel that they are worthwhile and helpful. Some therapists I know could persuade people to take winter holidays on Baffin Island. In the right therapist's hands, suggestion and persuasion are potent tools.

Therapy by suggestion is not a closed book. As Charles

Van Riper points out, stutterers can sometimes generate enough will-power to refuse to stutter for a short time. Nobody knows why it happens. A stutter cannot be cured by powerful self-persuasion alone, but stutterers can, at the end of successful therapy, be taught to resist the urge to stutter if avoidance of speaking is no longer a problem.

The stutterer is asked to read in unison with the fluent therapist, which he does very easily. Then the therapist stutters deliberately and challenges the patient to keep fluent. The stutterer must resist the therapist's suggestion to revert to old stuttering behaviour, and gradually the patient is persuaded to build up resistance to stress. In a similar way, delayed auditory feedback can be used to challenge the stutterer who has responded to therapy to keep fluent by will-power, even though the delayed sound tends to disrupt his fluency.[24]

This is, of course, very different from hypnosis, but there is a strong element of auto-suggestion. It does not support the views of people who say 'You can stop stuttering if you really want to,' because self-persuasion is only effective as part of other therapy.

Injudicious use of hypnosis to cure a stutter in the music-hall situation can be very damaging. If hypnosis is used at all it should follow a careful assessment of the stutterer by a qualified professional in a clinical situation. There are first-class hypnotists, but there are enough quacks to stock a duck farm.

The mind-benders: psychotherapy

PSYCHOANALYSIS

With the plethora of doubts about whether stuttering is caused by organic disorders, and the overwhelming amount of evidence that stuttering develops under social pressure and is maintained by anxieties about speaking and responses to stuttering cues, you would think that the psychoanalysts would have come up with more answers than they have. Most stutterers who received intensive therapy in the 1940s and 1950s found themselves at one time or another sitting opposite a Freudian psychiatrist who probed for evidence of neurosis by asking them personal questions about their childhood and love life. Few found it helped their speech. Earlier this century Brill had some success psychoanalyzing stutterers. Most of his sixty-nine patients responded, but the number of subsequent relapses was disappointing.[25] Such analysis is not a sure-fire cure.

These days fewer psychologists and psychiatrists carry out in-depth analyses to find the alleged neurotic causes of stuttering. There are many causes, all of them interacting, and a neurosis may or may not be one of them. The more common approach is to treat the stutterer as he is today, reduce his tensions and fears about speaking, modify negative attitudes, and teach him better ways of speaking.

You could expect that the daily trauma experienced to a greater or lesser degree by all severe stutterers would result in a definite 'stuttering personality,' even a neurotic one. In spite of a great deal of research, there is no real evidence of such an entity. According to H.R. Beech and Fay Fransella, 'If the stutterer has a unique personality pattern this would have been abundantly apparent by this time.'[26] It is hard for a psychotherapist to develop general principles and know precisely what to treat.

All psychotherapy encounters the problem that in order to treat the patient it is necessary to establish a dialogue, and stutterers find it so hard to speak that this can be remarkably difficult to achieve. Sometimes a stutterer can give misleading answers when he avoids difficult words. The classic story of the stutterer who, when asked by a waiter which salad dressing he wanted, said, 'Roque____, Roque____, Roque____, Thousand Islands,' gives a good example of word substitution. It is easier for most people with stutters to say 'Yes' than 'No.' If the patient tends to favour the response 'yes,' regardless of the question, the clinician is led into a maze of contradictions.

Nevertheless, psychoanalysis can help a stutterer respond to other therapy. Dealing with 'frozen feelings' is one area in which psychoanalysis is useful. Some stutterers are so adept at freezing their feelings when approaching a traumatic speaking situation that it becomes a way of life, spilling over into all their daily relationships. All people discipline their feelings to deal with their fears or they couldn't perform, but these emotions may catch up with them later. The trouble with people who stutter badly is that fears beset them so often that they discipline their feelings all the time and all too well. They never let go.

In 1943 a German fighter aircraft carried out a low-level, surprise attack on southeastern London during the lunch break. It had a persistent Spitfire on its tail. The intruder carried a 250-pound bomb beneath its fuselage, and the pilot dumped the explosives at random to reduce the plane's weight and increase its manoeuvrability. Tragically, the bomb landed on a primary school dining-room and blew many small children to pieces.

During the cleaning-up operation the workers did their job in silence, with expressionless, mask-like faces. The horror was too great for them to bear consciously, so they froze their feelings to allow them to do their jobs. In the evening they congregated in a nearby pub, where some just sat and stared into space over their untouched beers, while others openly wept. Each reacted in his own way. Those who accepted the pain of their emotions and wept were lucky, but some of those who remained frozen would never accept the penalty of their outraged feelings and would stash them away in locked closets in their minds. Some would have nightmares for many years unless they faced the horror squarely.

People who stutter deal with a multitude of lesser horrors and nightmares every day. If they continually store away and deny decades of unfelt pain it can make them very tense indeed. Psychoanalysis and counselling can help them to face their memories' spectres. Some people plagued by stuttering had such terrible experiences in their first years at school that they blot this period out of their minds. In-depth analysis can help them to accept the pain of the memory, see themselves as a whole, deal with any lingering deep resentment of their childhood tormentors, and get on with the speech therapy. Many adult stutterers dealt with their feelings themselves during their childhood, but for some it was too much to bear.

Psychological counselling can help those who stutter to deal with emotions (not necessarily neuroses) that come to the surface during other therapy. Stutterers respond in different ways to their disability, and some have deep-seated anger toward their parents, siblings, peers, or any segment of society that torments them. Sometimes they have good reason to be angry; but anger and bitterness, with violent verbal or even physical explosions, can become a way of life.

Psychotherapy can help a stutterer, or any other person, to manage anger in a productive, positive way. There are two schools of thought about how to do this. During the last decade many psychiatrists interpreted Freud's ideas to mean that all repression is bad and that to repress anger is dangerous to a person's mental health. These practitioners have encouraged people to express their hostility openly by screaming and throwing tantrums to 'let it all out'. Such quickie solutions to mankind's frustrations have in my opinion helped to generate our permissive, spoiled-brat society.

Carol Tavris has debunked the idea that it is wrong to control anger in her refreshing book *Anger: The Misunderstood Emotion.*[27] She points out that openly expressing violent anger and 'having it out' with your antagonist does not defuse the anger or make the exploder feel any better. There are better ways than fury and abuse to deal with injustice or insult.

The problem that many stutterers face is that they are not sufficiently fluent to use sharp-edged syntax as a defence against rudeness. In spite of this, some handle it very well. A burly man with a severe stutter went up to the counter of a coffee shop and blocked badly when he ordered a cup of coffee. A man who belonged to one of those charitable organizations that wear funny hats and help paraplegics was sitting nearby. He mimicked the stutterer's speech and laughed. The large stutterer went over to him and disfluently but calmly said, 'Why did you do that? Do you find my stutter funny? I don't. You people provide wheelchairs for the physically disabled and help the blind, deaf, and mentally retarded. What's so different about people who stutter? You wouldn't ridicule or mimic a person in a wheelchair.'

The man was shattered. He apologized, asked about the problem and how it was treated, and volunteered his help. He was just an ordinary, decent person programmed by Western society's mores to ridicule stuttering. The highly explosive situation was defused when the stutterer managed his intense anger in a constructive way.

Van Riper has said that deep psychoanalytic procedures 'have not been shown to be particularly effective with the stutterer,'[28] but Bloodstein has concluded that 'psychoanalytic treatment of stutterers to date ... appears to have been too good to permit us to reject this method summarily, and too poor as yet to warrant any substantial amount of satisfaction.'[29]

Whatever the initial cause, the stutterer may well have outgrown the original stimulus to stutter and left it far behind. His main problems are usually his anxiety about speech, society's reaction to his disability, and his inner and outer response to that reaction.

There are many ways of carrying out psychoanalysis, and it is not appropriate to describe them here. The earlier Freudian approaches seem to be giving way to behavioural methods. Now that some behaviourists are under attack for too close adherence to Skinnerian 'Operant Conditioning,' new avenues are being explored. Undoubtedly some stutterers have neuroses that need resolution by psychoanalysis, just as some blind people need psychiatric help; but most stutterers respond well to less detailed, short-term counselling and reduction of their sensitivity to stuttering cues and frustration. Gestalt therapy in various forms is used frequently as an adjunct to other therapy, so it is worth describing here.

GESTALT THERAPY
This approach is based on the principle that people are healthy when they are in touch with themselves and their surroundings. It emphasizes pattern, organization, and wholes, and involves the study of unanalysed personal experience rather than reflective introspection. The whole is looked on as quite different from the sum of the individual parts. The word 'gestalt' is hard to translate into English, but gestalten means a holistic pattern.

Gestalt therapy has been used to treat stutters by dealing with speech behaviour in relation to feelings and attitudes. The stutterer is made conscious of what he does when he stutters (stops breathing, purses the lips, lifts the tongue to the roof of the mouth), so that he can accept personal responsibility for the way he speaks and realize that, with guidance, he can modify his stuttering behaviour by continuing airflow and reducing lip and tongue tensions.

Many stutterers feel that there is a perverse little manikin inside them that makes them stutter, when in fact the stutterer himself is responsible for his stutter. He is shown that he can learn to choose whether he tenses lips and tongue or approaches speech in a gentle manner, stops breathing or continues his airflow. He can learn to choose between stuttering and fluency.

In order to be responsible for the way he speaks and to modify his speech patterns, he must stay in contact with his audience and not go off into the detached trance with which so many blocked stutterers remove themselves mentally from the intolerable situation. He is shown how to focus on the solution rather than the problem. A stutterer can't focus on anything if he has floated off into the protective never-never land of the severely disfluent. Gestalt therapy helps the stutterer to take more risks by testing unfamiliar ways of speaking in many different situations.

Gestalt therapy guides the stutterer to be aware of his conflict about wanting to speak yet not wanting to because of his stutter, and to stay in touch with his feelings, his audience, and his surroundings. The therapy deals with anxiety by persuading the stutterer to stop worrying about what is going to happen (don't anticipate the day's traumatic speaking situations) and to direct his attention and energies to present problems and their solutions. The over-all goal is to keep the stutterer in touch with his feelings and surroundings, and to modify attitudes that increase or reinforce his abnormal speech.[30]

Therapy similar to the Gestalt approach is used in most speech clinics, although not always under a Gestalt label. Treatment of avoidances, conflicts, awareness, and anxiety are the core of many modern therapies. Helping the stutterer to stay in contact, to understand what he does when he stutters, and to realize that he can choose to use the better speaking techniques offered by the therapists is important if the stutterer is to gain any freedom from the fear that is part of the problem. Supportive psychotherapy helps to clear the clutter from the stutterer's workbench so he can get on with the business of reconstructing his speech.

CONDITIONING AND FLUENCY SHAPING
Conditioning therapy is more favoured by clinicians than by the general public, who tend to associate it with brainwashing. Nevertheless new conditioning techniques are having great success.

A person with a stutter is conditioned to respond to numerous cues that trigger stuttering. One stutterer I knew in the Armed Forces savagely blocked whenever he saw a floral fabric because whenever he stuttered a sadistic schoolteacher had draped him over a chair covered with the fabric and beaten him for lazy speech, allegedly to help him. Most stuttering cues (particular sounds or words) are less dramatic, and it is fair to assume that what has been conditioned can be deconditioned by appropriate therapy. If an experimental rat can be taught to press a lever to obtain food or avoid pain, surely a person who stutters can be taught to speak in a normal way. Therapy that uses conditioning can reduce stutterers' sensitivities to cues, anxiety, and frustration. Even so, it is not as straightforward as many people think.

I am aware that many of my cues are indirect. Even pictures of objects or types of places or people associated with traumatic stuttering in the past can trigger a stuttering phase. Just the sight of a building can set me off. This became apparent when a clinician screened a series of slides and asked me to talk about them. Pictures of lecture halls, telephones, police cars, adolescents, customs officials, and people chatting socially, gave me great trouble until I was desensitized by repeated exposure. I didn't fear any of these images, but past associations made them trigger my stuttering. I was conditioned to respond to them and had to be desensitized systematically.

A classic example of indirect conditioning is the 'Albert's fear of furry objects' case. In the early 1920s a small American child called Albert was conditioned to be scared of furry objects by first frightening him with the noise made by striking a steel bar and then pairing a furry object with the noise. Although Albert was initially scared of the noise and responded to it, he later responded fearfully to furry objects without the noise. I can't help wondering what happened to Albert and speculating about how many furry objects scared him in later life.[31]

The conditioning techniques used to remove old bad habits and instil new and better ones mostly come under the broad heading of 'operant conditioning,' the principle of which is that when you behave in a certain way and there are consequences, these consequences influence your future behaviour.

When the consequences involve a reward (positive reinforcement), the behaviour is likely to be repeated. If the behaviour results in punishment (negative reinforcement), the behaviour is often avoided or weakened. A punishment following a form of behaviour can be made to reduce the behaviour, which is the principle underlying civil retribution for acts against society. Behaviour that removes the penalty or prevents it from occurring can be strengthened.[32]

The earlier work on operant conditioning tended to skim over innate factors like genes and the urge to seek novelty and assumed that any animal could be conditioned to do anything. Although this is now questioned, there is no doubt that experience affects fear and our responses to it. A subject's fear can be reduced if the feared situation is repeated without penalty (a technique used in speech therapy under the heading of 'desensitization') or if it is apparent that certain behaviour can end or prevent pain.

Whatever reduces a stutterers' fear of speaking has potential as a therapeutic tool, and operant conditioning, with its rewards and punishments for speech behaviour, has been used to improve stutterers' fluency. Rewards and punishments seem to have worked at least temporarily for some, but I am glad that it is one form of therapy I missed. There are more than enough penalties for stuttering already.

The effects of operant conditioning on stuttering were studied by Flanagan and his colleagues.[33] They subjected three patients to a punishing 105-decibel noise every time they blocked, and the subjects' disfluency was reduced considerably. It was also found that when the noise was con-

tinuous except when switched off briefly if a patient stuttered, stuttering increased. In other words the patients who
stuttered became more fluent to avoid the noise penalty in the
first case, and then stuttered to get subsequent peace and
quiet in the second case. The speech responses were thought
to be due to the consequences of stuttering – noise or silence.

Martin and Siegel found that when stuttering was penalized by electrical shocks from electrodes strapped to the patient's wrist, disfluency was markedly reduced. The improvement continued in the clinic without the shocks if the electrodes were simply attached, but the speech broke down
when they were removed. One patient remained fluent when
he wore a plain wrist-strap reminiscent of the punitive electrodes. In another situation a patient who stuttered became
temporarily more fluent when he was simultaneously shocked
and exposed to a blue light each time he stuttered. His fluency
increased with the blue light alone, but the stuttering returned
when both electrodes and the blue light were removed. Verbal
punishment and rewards ('Not good' or 'Good') were also effective in reducing stuttering in the clinic, and a simple wrist
strap to remind the stutterer to say each word as fluently as
possible helped to maintain fluency.[34] These studies were
research rather than therapy. They aimed at studying the effects of rewards and penalties.

In 1969, the Speech Foundation of America sponsored a
conference at Montego Bay, Jamaica, to discuss the use of
operant conditioning in stuttering therapy. The participants
included such respected therapists as Joseph G. Sheehan and
Charles Van Riper, who revolutionized stuttering therapy in
North America, as well as professors of other university
speech departments.

The experts were cautious about the desirability of using
punishment to achieve fluency. As Van Riper reminded the
participants, 'These stuttering clients of ours are not Skinnerian pigeons hatched from laboratory eggs. They are not
Pavlovian dogs suspended from experimental frames. They
are subject to other controls more powerful than those we
can mobilize in the therapy room. Stutterers come to us with
long histories of past conditioning ... Behaviour therapists
have difficulty working with stutterers.' In similar vein,

Joseph Sheehan asked, 'Why should children stutter when the behaviour is apparently more punished than rewarded?' If punishment were an effective stuttering deterrent there would be few stutterers in Western society.[35]

Conditioning in benign forms is widely used today under the title of 'Fluency Shaping Therapy.' Operant conditioning and programming principles, with the reward-punishment aspects well hidden, are used in this therapy, which differs from therapies that attempt to treat the stutterer as a whole person. Fluency shaping therapy takes a direct approach. It assumes that the stutterer makes the sounds of speech incorrectly and that reasons for this are beside the point. Researchers of this school of thought have carefully examined what a stutterer does incorrectly and look upon stuttering as part of a speech spectrum ranging from severe disfluency to normal speech. The therapy is designed to push the speech toward the normal end of this spectrum by carefully graded exercises that emphasize the control of speech rate, gentle initial approaches (easy onset) to sounds, and prolongation of words to achieve fluency within the clinic. Later the techniques are transferred to everyday life.[36]

This technique was used by Ronald L. Webster, of Hollins College, Virginia, and his innovative approach evolved after a series of experimental programs. The earlier programs used delayed auditory feedback to achieve fluency, and the later schemes tried to overcome the fact that the stutterer tended to use the clinician as a crutch. The final treatment consisted of teaching the patient how to handle single sounds, followed by whole words, transition from word to word, prolongation, and an impersonal monitoring system.

This system minimizes the frequency with which the therapist must tell the stutterer what to do next. When the patient speaks correctly, a light flashes to indicate that he can move on to other exercises. If the light does not flash, the stutterer repeats the sound or word until it is correct. The frequency of disfluencies is recorded to assess improvement.

All tasks are carefully graded, and even the sounds are ranked according to difficulty. Vowels are the easiest; vowel-like consonants ('l,' 'r,' 'y,' and 'w') are a little harder; fricatives ('f' and 's') harder still; and stop-consonants (the plosives 'p,' 'b,' and 'd') hardest of all. The aim is to instruct the stutterer to start his sounds gently, handle 'silent' consonants correctly, and increase the duration of sounds.

Early in the therapy the duration of sounds is very exaggerated, but the prolongation is reduced until the rate of speaking is about 100 words or more per minute, which is slow but socially acceptable. The transfer of these techniques to everyday life was found to be unusually good, and positive results were obtained after only forty to sixty hours in the clinic. A set of twenty patients aged from eight to fifty-two years responded remarkably well. After treatment, nineteen reported better speech. Only one person felt that his stutter was the same. After therapy many of the stutterers talked more, as you would expect, were better able to take part in a wider range of social activities, and found their work easier to handle.[37]

The Webster or Hollins method[38] has aroused considerable interest and is now an important component of many programs. It may not help stutterers who hide their stuttering and refuse to stutter openly. The Webster method can greatly help the more open stutterers.

I recently revisited my old *alma mater*, the Royal Ottawa Hospital, and was greeted by the sound of slow, melodic chanting, as though somebody were intoning mantras. Closer inspection revealed the patients sitting in front of electronic boxes with flashing lights, holding all their syllables for one or two seconds. There was great emphasis on the gentle approach to words.

The sessions were remarkably relaxed. The highlight of the visit was when the group chanted 'Happy Birthday to You' holding each syllable for two or three seconds. Try it some time!

The well-known Monterey Program for stutterers employed by the Behavioural Sciences Institute in Monterey, California, also involves conditioning. It uses two approaches: GILCU (gradual increase in length and complexity of utterances) and delayed auditory feedback (DAF).

The patient progresses step by step from easy words to hard words. If he is fluent he is rewarded ('Good!'). If he stutters he is penalized ('Stop! Do it again.') He graduates from single words, to word pairs, to triplets, and then to whole sentences. Reading is followed by monologues and then conversation. He learns to transfer his fluency to the outside world. When patients find this approach to fluency difficult, DAF is used, and the goal is 0.5 stuttered word or less per minute for a period of five minutes. Results have been promising but maintenance of the improvement is still a problem.[39]

A clinician must decide which type of treatment is suitable for particular patients. It is usual to carry out an analysis of the patient's stuttering behaviour and engage in trial therapy before deciding whether or not fluency shaping therapy is the right approach. The speech is recorded on tapes, and the number of words or syllables stuttered per minute counted. Rate of speaking in words per minute may also be estimated. The severity of stuttering can be assessed in several ways, and therapists use various scales for rating the severity of stuttering. The clinician tries to assess the stutterer's attitudes about himself and his speech, and to what extent the disability is affecting his life, work, and happiness. She may use an informal, qualitative approach or a more precise, quantitative rating.[40]

The trial therapy assesses how well the patient responds to therapeutic procedures by speaking slowly and prolonging words. If the stutterer does not appear to be plagued by strong emotions about his speech, is accepted by family and peers, doesn't find that the stutter interferes a great deal with his life, doesn't disguise his stuttering, and is comfortable with using prolonged speech, he is probably a candidate for treatment by fluency shaping procedures. If the stutterer has been heavily penalized by society for his disability, is not readily accepted at home or school, hides his stutter, is uncomfortable with slow prolonged speech, and is obviously unhappy with or constrained by his impediment, he may respond better to therapy that treats the whole person, which may help him deal with his anxieties. Sometimes a combination of fluency shaping therapy and other methods is appropriate.[41]

In fluency shaping therapy there is little need for the stutterer to try to perform tasks that arouse great fear, because the approach is carefully structured. The therapists for this treatment are also relatively easy to train. One disadvantage is that the method requires the stutterer to speak in an abnormally slow, prolonged fashion until fluency is achieved in the clinic, and some stutterers find this both objectionable and remarkably difficult. The structured and more impersonal approach is less interesting for the therapist than techniques with more personal involvement.

Stuttering modifiers

Stuttering modification therapy is based on the idea that a person stutters because he struggles with or avoids disfluencies, feared words and sounds, and feared situations. The therapy is designed to reduce avoidances, anxieties about speaking, and negative attitudes about speech, and to help the stutterer *modify* his disfluency. The stutterer is taught to avoid fighting his blocks, to smooth out his stutter, to reduce tension, and to stutter more slowly in a relaxed and deliberate way. The therapy has a considerable psychotherapeutic content in addition to speech modification and, in contrast to fluency shaping therapy, attempts to treat the person as a whole instead of dealing exclusively with faulty speech habits.

A great deal of this therapy was developed at the University of Iowa Speech Clinic and at Western Michigan University. It is sometimes called the 'Iowa Method.'

Stuttering modification therapy in its many forms has revolutionized speech therapy in North America and its influence has been felt all over the world. During the 1920s it was all too clear that people with stutters were not responding well to psychoanalysis or to such conventional speech therapies as relaxation and distraction. Most of the patients relapsed. Carl Emil Seashore, a well known psychologist, who was Dean of the Graduate College at the University of Iowa, recognized the need for a better scientific understanding of speech and hearing disorders. In 1927, he selected Lee Edward Travis as Director of the Iowa Speech Clinic with a mandate to focus the skills of several university departments on hearing and speech problems, to establish a firm scientific basis, and to develop a program on a wider front than before.[42]

Following Travis's appointment there was a period of intense speculation about the origins of stuttering and experimentation with methods of treatment. Techniques evolved that tried both to reduce fears and avoidances and to change speaking patterns. Patients were taught to stutter openly with minimal abnormality and without fear.

Bryng Bryngelson, Wendell Johnson, Charles Van Riper, and Joseph Sheehan were the key figures who brought about this revolution in speech therapy. In the 1930s Bryngelson taught his patients to repeat sounds deliberately in a controlled way (voluntary controlled repetition, or VCR), and to stop avoiding stuttering and become objective about it. He stressed the group approach and encouraged the stutterers to take the techniques out of the clinic into real-life situations.

On a different tack, Wendell Johnson used voluntary controlled repetition to reduce the stutterer's caution about speaking, and to teach him to speak without tension until the disfluency resembled the pauses and hesitations of a normal speaker. Johnson felt strongly that the way a stutterer perceives his speech makes him stutter. He tried to make people with stutters responsible for their own speech instead of blaming their problem on something beyond their control. I have often said to myself that I block because my airflow ceases and my tongue rises in my mouth and becomes inflexible, but this is nonsense. My *tongue* doesn't rise; I *make* it rise, for some reason or other. I stutter because of what *I* do, not because of what my tongue decides to do. This may appear to be mere semantics, but the 'General Semantics Theory' of Polish philosopher, mathematician, and engineer Alfred Korzybski played a major role in Wendell Johnson's methods.

This theory is concerned with the relationships between the language people use and the way they think and act. Wendell Johnson drew upon Korzybski's ideas about why education, politics, and philosophy have progressed so slowly compared with science. Korzybski felt that science had progressed because precise information had been passed from one generation to another in such a manner that what was said matched the facts. In contrast, other human affairs have developed on the chaotic basis of inheritance of false but unquestioned assumptions, traditions, habits, attitudes, beliefs, and doctrines. As he said, 'It is not an exaggeration that it (language) enslaves us through the mechanism of semantic reaction,' and he suggested that the structure of our language affects the nervous system.

Johnson applied this theory to the stutterer's false assumptions that any disfluency is socially unacceptable, that speaking is difficult, and that stuttering is caused by something (other than himself) that stops him speaking. His therapy tried to dispel these false assumptions by letting the patient observe what happened when he spoke fluently. He could see and hear both that he could be fluent and that normal speakers could be disfluent. Johnson's therapy involved a great deal of group discussion of the stutterer's perception of his abnormal speech, and the patient was encouraged to assume that there was no uncontrollable organic or emotional reason why he should be abnormally disfluent.[43]

These approaches helped many stutterers, but in spite of the emphasis on adopting new attitudes and using better speaking techniques in real-life situations, stutterers still tended to relapse. It is difficult to keep an eye on your attitudes and mode of speaking all the time during a working day. Old fears about speaking and well-established stuttering cues all too frequently penetrate the chinks in the stutterer's newly acquired armour of objectivity.

Charles Van Riper established a speech clinic at Western Michigan University, carried out numerous experiments on stuttering, varied the therapy, and kept long-term records to discover how well patients maintained their speech improvement after therapy. His approach included elements of the Iowa method (like reducing anxiety about stuttering and modifying stuttering behaviour by a patient's analysis of his own speech) and emphasized the need for stutterers to stutter fluently rather than to try to speak completely fluently and normally. He tried to minimize the abnormality without completely removing it.[44]

Van Riper's stuttering modification methods have been

remarkably successful. Five years after treatment, about 50 per cent of the stutterers he treated were very fluent, didn't exhibit fear of their stuttering, and didn't avoid hard words or difficult speaking situations. Many other patients greatly improved their speech and developed attitudes that enabled them to live more normal lives. The carry-over into everyday life of the speech improvement resulting from Van Riper's modification of the Iowa method was much better than with previous therapies.

Van Riper looked upon a stutter as a self-perpetuating, learned behaviour, regardless of the original causes. He felt that this behaviour arose from fearful anticipation and frustration resulting from past episodes of abnormal disfluency. He attempted to teach patients to stutter more normally. Although he used voluntary controlled repetition for speech exercises, he emphasized the use of smooth, prolonged speech that simplified the stuttering and made the speech more continuous. Prolongation of sound is widely used in modern therapy.

The technique was not easy to learn, and the stutterer's inclination to approach difficult words with pre-set lips and tongue and anxious anticipation still tended to disrupt the continuity. Van Riper realized that the short period of expectancy before saying a word was important and developed ways a stutterer could respond to this expectancy by preforming a better set of lip and tongue positions in place of the old, destructive sets. When a stutterer expected difficulty, he was to place his lips and tongue at rest and say the first sound so that it led into the next sound. Voice and airflow were started immediately. Van Riper worked to alter the stutterer's preparatory sets so that he could stutter more fluently.

Although this method gave good results, there were still problems. The stutterer had to watch his speech closely all the time and sometimes didn't change his approach to words as he should have done. To overcome this, Van Riper taught stutterers to pull out of their blocks with smooth prolongation. Again, this worked well, but stutterers still tended to get firmly entrapped in a block before they could organize their speech to pull out of it, so Van Riper developed methods of cancelling blocks. When the stutterer's speech stuck because he didn't use prolongation and pull-outs correctly, he was taught to pause, examine his feelings and speech behaviour, and try again.

The new techniques of preparatory sets, pulling out of blocks, and pausing when difficulties were encountered constitute the core of Van Riper's therapy, which also deals effectively with a stutterer's guilt, hostility, penalties, frustrations, fears of words and situations, morale, low self-esteem, and misconceptions.

His therapy does not involve psychoanalysis. Nevertheless, it is a psychotherapeutic approach that takes into account the many facets of the stuttering syndrome, reinforcing those that help a stutterer and removing those that make him lose control of his speech. Van Riper realized that penalties, frustration, anxiety, guilt, hostility, situation fears, word-phonetic fears, and the importance of what was being said could all make a stutter worse. In contrast, good morale, a strong ego, and past experience of fluency could improve a stutter. He designed individual therapies to reduce the factors that make a stutter worse and strengthen those that make it better, recognizing that the importance of individual factors varies considerably from one stutterer to another.[45]

A therapist treating young stuttering children with Van Riper's methods concentrates on a whole complex of things: reducing penalties; reducing a child's frustration; building up his tolerance to frustration; reducing anxiety, guilt, and hostility; releasing forbidden feelings; counselling parents individually and in groups; reducing the stresses and demands of communication; and increasing the amount of fluency a child experiences so that he can respond to it. In some children it is necessary to improve their self-regard and morale. When a child becomes aware of his stuttering, and the repetitions and abnormal prolongations impede his communication, treatment of frustration will become a necessary part of the therapy. He may not fear speech as much as older stutterers, and a child's stutter is far less complex than the full-blown, severe stutter of an adult, but his abnormal disfluency can make his life difficult.

There are a great many ways of treating children's stutters along these lines. If the child is treated when very young, his chances of achieving socially acceptable fluency are high. It is not possible to discuss all the techniques but some of those described by Van Riper in his excellent books, *Speech Correction: Principles and Methods*, 5th edition (1972), and *Treatment of Stuttering* (1973), are of particular interest.

A child finds it difficult to express his feelings about his speech and himself and, when he attempts to do so, he is all too often penalized or ignored by an impatient adult. Play therapy lets the child either say or act out his deep feelings and needs to a caring therapist. The therapist, in the role of a new parent, helps the child to recognize his fears and desires so that he can re-evaluate them.[46] The slightly different approach of 'Creative Dramatics' encourages children to improvise a play, invent the dialogue, and select parts to give them the opportunity to express their intense feelings.

Van Riper quotes a children's play about King Midas and his Golden Touch. One of the children, a boy, acted the part of King Midas by portraying him as a cruel man who shouted at the servants, hit the table, and ordered impossible things. The plot of the story was lost in the ranting and raving. When asked why he played the role in this way, the boy said he thought King Midas was a cruel man, as mean as his teacher.[47] Many people who stutter will recognize an echo of their own early experiences with impatient teachers at school.

The advantage of dramatics is that the child can express himself in front of a sympathetic group, and the method is used as a back-up to play therapy. It is not regarded as a suitable approach for children whose contact with reality is tenuous and who tend to fantasize and play roles , but Van Riper did find creative dramatics useful in resolving problems of sibling rivalry, teasing by playmates, and dealing with bullies.

Some children either do not respond well to the co-ordinated approaches of Van Riper and proponents of the Iowa method or have parents and teachers who cannot or will not modify their damaging responses to the children's abnormal speech. Desensitization therapy, which is used in different ways with both children and adult stutterers, teaches the stutterer to become less sensitive to the rejections, impatience, or worse by adapting to these adversities.

When parents are effectively counselled and ease the pressures on a stuttering child at home, the child may lower his level of tolerance. This can be disastrous in the classroom. The therapist helps the child to adopt and feel a basic fluency and then exposes him to increasing pressures of the type that precipitate his stuttering. As soon as the child shows signs of impending disfluency by increased rigidity and jerkiness, the therapist goes back to the basic fluency. This is repeated and gradually the child is able to tolerate more and more disruption. In these sessions, the child's fluency is carefully maintained under pressure and the effects seem to carry over into situations outside the clinic. Obviously, it requires a sensitive and skilful therapist and the trust of the child.

When treating a confirmed stutterer with many years of abnormal disfluency, Van Riper took into account anxieties about particularly difficult words and speaking situations. The adult stutterer's fears about words and situations tend to overshadow other factors – like penalties, frustrations, anxiety, guilt, and hostility – that increase stuttering. Many therapists focus on treating these word and situation fears and on strengthening the stutterer's morale and experiences of fluency.

Stuttering modification therapy and Van Riper's extension of it are widely used today in North America. The details vary, but in general the therapist makes a total attack on all the factors that increase stuttering. The adult stutterer is not penalized for stuttering, which is encouraged so long as it is done in a prolonged, fluent manner. Every attempt is made to reduce the penalties a stutterer has incurred because of his stuttering. The effects of frustration are reduced by permitting the patient to stutter, and efforts are made to build up his tolerance to frustration. Group discussions help the patient to share his experiences, good and bad, with others, to air his feelings, and to act out conflicts. Together with professional counselling and, if necessary, psychotherapy, this helps the adult stutterer to reduce his problems of anxiety and guilt.

The stuttering modification approach is complex and contains a large element of psychotherapy and counselling. It is rooted in many qualitative assumptions, and the therapy requires considerable skill on the part of the therapist – far more than that required to prescribe the pills and potions upon which modern medicine relies so heavily. A good stuttering modification therapist shares a stutterer's fears and frustrations and helps him to deal with them. She may also incorporate psychotherapy and fluency shaping to achieve the planned goals.

An eclectic form of therapy, including stuttering modification with its echoes of Bryngelson, Johnson, Van Riper, and Sheehan, together with some of the elements of fluency shaping is described in detail in *Clinical Manual for the Comprehensive Stuttering Program* (1984), by Einer Boberg and Deborah Kully of the Department of Speech Pathology and Audiology at the University of Alberta in Edmonton. Their supplementary *Client Manual* will help patients understand what is ahead of them.[48]

The Iowa developments led to an appreciation of the stutterer as a person. The approach is more humane than the regimentation and browbeating associated with so many of the earlier therapies. The stutterer is led to his solution rather than bludgeoned into temporary fluency by threats and criticism. The fact that some of the originators of these new, humane approaches – among them Charles Van Riper – were themselves stutterers increases the confidence of people who stutter in the techniques. Doubtless their success results from these clinicians' deep understanding of how a stutterer perceives his speech, himself, and the world around him. A person is likely to be better equipped to dispel the barrier of a stutterer's glass tower when he has been imprisoned within such a tower himself.

A problem facing all therapists is that of logistics. There are many millions of people in the world who stutter. By no means all of them come for therapy, even in North America and Europe; even so, in the more affluent Western societies there are more applications for treatment than the clinics can handle.

Stuttering modification therapy often takes one or more years and, because of the necessarily close relationship between the therapist and the patient, classes tend to be small and the turnover slow. It is not a therapy for mass application. Fluency shaping therapy takes only a month or so, apart from later maintenance. It has a much more rapid turnover and is more suitable for the treatment of large numbers of people.

The short-term success of some therapies, particularly conditioning therapies, has led to an almost evangelical attitude in some clinicians. Comments like, 'My therapy is the only one that works,' and 'All other therapies are bunk,' occasionally appear like graffiti on the clinical fabric. Even in the newsletters of stutterers' self-help organizations, professionals and near-professionals acridly denounce each other's views. Like most evangelists, their hearts are in the right place. They want to help people and feel strongly that their way to salvation is best. The ones to look out for are the speech-pathology equivalents of those articulate, hard-eyed, grey-suited evangelists on television who want to save your soul and reduce your bank balance at the same time.

In spite of all the difficulties, the incidence of successful therapy is increasing. Whether it will level off in the face of our ignorance about the causes of the malady remains to be seen. A better understanding of the neurology of stuttering should help to remove the remaining barriers. In the past decade a vast amount of research on stuttering has been carried out, and information is accumulating at an incredible rate. It just needs a genius to put it all together.

Will the benefits of speech therapy last forever?

This is the knottiest and most frustrating question of all. It all comes under the heading 'maintenance,' a word that causes therapists and stutterers alike many sleepless nights, heartaches, and even nightmares.

Some patients with relatively mild stutters go to a clinic, learn new speech techniques, and apply them in real life. No trouble at all. They never look back as they fluently chatter their way through life.

Then there are those like myself with stuttering so firmly riveted into their psychological bulkheads that it needs a therapeutic blow-torch to loosen it and let the words flow.

I had been in the audio-visual lab most of a hot summer's day. Even with television cameras trained on me, my therapist hadn't been able to shake my beautifully controlled speech. It was solid as the Rock of Gibraltar. A telephone assignment had been tough, but apart from a little tension it went remarkably well. Four years of therapy were yielding their fruit.

Thirsty after all the talking, I went to my usual watering hole where they keep a good line in draught beer. Full of confidence I sat at my usual glossy plastic table and signalled my favourite waitress, thinking of the frosted, frothy tankard ahead. When her pencil was poised over her pad I happily started to ask for my beer. I say 'started,' but that was as far as it went. Not a sound came out. Not a whisper. Just the faint gagging noise of a massive block which wafted my attention aloft into the never-never land of a stutterer's detachment, where he can think of anything except how to get out of the mess he's in.

I gradually fought my way out of the detachment and at last managed to cancel the block with a long sigh of released air. Smiling ruefully at the waitress I said with no effort at all, 'All I'm trying to do is order a darned draught beer!' We both laughed.

Back to the drawing board for another year or more.

Maintenance is so important that there's a whole 284-page book about it, *The Maintenance of Fluency* (1981), edited by Einer Boberg of the University of Alberta. It describes the views of the world's foremost speech pathologists about how to design therapies with longer lasting benefits. [49]

The sad fact is that many people who stutter go for treatment, revel in their new-found fluency in the clinic, and then face the heartbreak of a relapse. Relapse rates are much lower than they were a few years ago, but they are still uncomfortably high.

In order to maintain his better fluency a person with a severe stutter must practise the new way of speaking for about one hour every day, try it out in new situations, be philosophical about failures and encouraged by successes, and return to the clinic periodically for reinforcement of the methods and removal of any sloppiness. Many find it a great help to participate in self-help groups that will monitor speech.

It needs courage, discipline, and determination, and not all people have the inner resources.

At one time I practised speaking techniques for eight hours every day, soon cutting it to five, and eventually down to one. At this level of reinforcement I kept fairly fluent.

Since then my speech has been generally better, but I've become sloppy and lazy, finding it hard to think about my speech all the time for years on end. Consequently I still fall into verbal traps. However, the earlier therapy helps me to pull out of the chasms of major speech blocks. I no longer go into the free fall of tense silence that I used to experience many times every day.

Yes, the improvement achieved at the clinic can be maintained by many people, but for some it is not an easy road.

Which treatments are most successful?

Anybody embarking on the painful voyage of intensive therapy needs some idea of the chances of success. It is not possible to generalize, because so much depends on the type of stutter the patient has, his personality, the effort he is willing to make, and the skill of the therapist. Nevertheless there is evidence that some therapists are more successful than others.

Gavin Andrews and his colleagues at the University of New South Wales, Sydney, Australia, used a statistical method, meta-analysis, to compare the effectiveness of several techniques, including breath control (airflow), attitude therapy, biofeedback, desensitization, gently approaching sounds and words (gentle onset), prolonged speech, rhythm, and slow speaking.[50] They concluded that for adults prolonged speech and gentle onset to sounds and words were more effective than any other techniques in both the short and the long term. Rhythmic therapy had good initial results, but the benefit tended to fade considerably. Prolongation and gentle onset are combined with speaking slowly in many therapy programs, for example in Webster's fluency shaping and the Iowa school's stuttering modification.

This does not mean that the other techniques are useless. Biofeedback and desensitization are both in their infancy and may prove to be valuable therapeutic tools, and attitude therapy helps a great many stutterers.

Andrews and his colleagues feel that the clinical evidence does not support the widely held idea that stuttering is ill-understood and difficult to treat. A great deal is known about the possible causes of stuttering, the different methods of treatment, and the likely outcome. The facts are there; the only mystery is how to fit them together. The chances that therapy will improve a stutterer's speech are high, and getting better every year. We are no longer in the Dark Ages of stuttering therapy; the prognosis for people who stutter is encouraging.

If a stutterer can't get any therapy at all, therefore, it seems that the best thing he can do is speak very slowly, prolong his words, and approach the beginnings of words as gently as possible.

SIX

Where can a stutterer get the right kind of help?

'To help all created things, that is the measure of our responsibility; to be helped by all, that is the measure of our hope.'

Gerald Vaun

Stutterers who refuse to participate in formal therapy are likely to read this book. They usually read all books on stuttering, good and bad, that they can get their hands on, searching for a glimmer of light at the end of their handicap's tunnel. Doubtless they will read the menu of treatments and be tempted to try out rhythmic and other distractive methods. They will be delighted with the initial results and shattered when their speech falls apart.

This is *not* a self-help book and should not be used as such. Different types of stutterers need different types of treatment, and an effective, systematic approach is best designed by a competent professional after a full assessment of the problem. Some methods, even the good ones, can have a profound emotional impact, and it is useful to have psychological counsellors available to help smooth the therapy path and pick up the pieces when necessary. Going it alone with speech therapy without professional guidance is as wise as choosing your own pills in a pharmacy. By sheer luck you may get relief, but the side effects could be devastating.

Finding the best clinic

If an adult stutterer decides to seek help, what does he do? The obvious step is to go to the family doctor who will refer him to the nearest rehabilitation centre in a large hospital. Most rehabilitation departments provide treatment for a variety of communication disorders, including stutters. For some people this is the best approach, but there are several difficulties. A large rehabilitation centre is usually in a city. Since the early, intensive part of therapy involves regular visits, people living in outlying districts find it hard to attend and persist with the treatment. Some hospitals offer intensive courses of two or three weeks followed by less frequent visits. Even if the treatment is free, the sessions involve spending money on accommodation and meals. Over a period of four years I spent more than $5,000 (Canadian funds) on travel alone. A major problem is the amount of time the therapy takes. I used up a great deal of my leave going to and from the clinics.

Many of the speech therapists working on their own in small towns and rural areas are highly competent, but they are not likely to have the audio-visual equipment and electronic monitors that play such an important part in modern speech therapy. The smaller hospitals' budgets are limited, and these centres do not usually have on staff a psychologist who specializes in speech disorders to help when the going gets tough. Smaller facilities are excellent for subsequent speech maintenance, but may be less effective for initial therapy than hospitals with more resources.

The family physician may refer a patient who stutters to an unsuitable rehabilitation centre. There are good centres for treating stuttering and bad centres. Even an excellent family physician may not be well informed about stuttering or in a position to assess the quality of the treatment. A centre that deals with communication disorders in general may not have much experience of treating stuttering.

What does the stutterer do? He should do a little leg-work to find out about speech therapy in his own area before he sees his family physician. This is not usually as difficult as it sounds. Most countries have speech and hearing associations, which are good starting points. In the United States, the Speech Foundation of America (152 Lombardy Road, Memphis, Tennessee 38111), a non-profit charitable organization, provides guidance for stutterers and parents. This organization publishes and sells first-class, low-cost publications on stuttering and its early recognition and treatment written in non-technical language. The American Speech-Language-Hearing Association (ASHA) and its consumer branch can also be approached for information.[1] The Canadian equivalent is the Canadian Speech and Hearing Association (Royal York Hotel, Convention Mezzanine, 100 Front Street, Toronto, Ontario M5J 1E3), which is the parent body for its provincial satellites.[2] There are similar organizations in most countries. Most associations will answer enquiries about where therapy is available and which are the main centres, and some may indicate where progressive therapy can be found.

It is a great help to talk to other stutterers who have been treated at the different clinics. Sometimes you can find them in self-help groups. Other stutterers can often tell you whether a therapist is an inflexible authoritarian bully, or supportive, flexible, and progressive. Anyone who says they can *cure* the stutter should be looked upon with suspicion, because no responsible therapist will make that claim. An indication that a clinic relies completely on relaxation, medication, rhythmics, or distractions is also reason for caution. Evidence that a program involves a methodical rehabilitation of a stutterer's speech, using a flexible team approach with the stutterer helping others, and includes a follow-up program for speech maintenance is a good sign that the therapy is in touch with modern developments.

At this point a chat with the physician is needed. Some doctors may resent the fact that a patient has done research, but most will be glad to discuss the pros and cons of different types of therapy in the area. When the stutterer has been referred to a speech centre for assessment, he can meet the therapists and discuss the approach with them. They will know better than the stutterer what combination of treatments he needs, but at least he can assess whether or not they are using outmoded techniques that give short-term relief. Blind faith in any treatment is neither necessary nor desirable, but confidence in the therapist and the therapy is vital. There is no harm at all in going over the strategy of the therapy. The reluctance of some doctors to discuss with patients their prognosis and treatment is, or should be, obsolete.

If the stutterer likes what he hears, he needs the time, money, and motivation to embark upon the therapy, and the guts and discipline to persist with it over a period of months or even years. If he is seeking therapy he probably has good motives. He may be tired of society's rejection, discrimination, and cruelty, weary of not being able to participate in class discussions, or just interested in making more friends. One stutterer entered therapy after a horrendous session in court, during which the lawyer and judge had been unsympathetic about and critical of his disability. Many come for treatment only when they are desperate for help.

Self-treatment

The majority of stutterers do not have access to good speech therapy and cannot spare the time, money, and energy needed to attend clinics regularly. They have to rely on their own resources. This is not desirable, but it is a fact.

If a stutterer decides to treat his own disability with the help of his family and friends, he would be well advised to read Malcolm Fraser's booklet *To the Stutterer* and his excellent guide to self-treatment, sponsored and published by the Speech Foundation of America, *Self-Therapy for the Stutterer*.[3] The latter is endorsed by respected therapist Charles Van Riper, is based upon the treatments evolved by the Iowa and Michigan schools, and is easy to understand. The author assumes that stuttering is a form of behaviour that can be changed and describes how to analyse stuttering, control blocks, and face up to fears. Speaking slowly, using the easy-onset approach to words, stuttering openly and easily, ceasing to avoid situations or to substitute words, maintaining eye contact, using voluntary controlled repetition, cancellation, and easy pulling out from blocks are all advocated. All the elements of good modern therapy are there, but a speech therapist and a psychologist to encourage and guide the stutterer are absent. Other useful books are Ainsworth's *Counselling Stutterers*[4] and Irwin's *Stammering: Practical Help for All Ages*.[5]

Self-treatment is likely to be a long, hard road with many false starts and pitfalls and possibly periods of great distress and disappointment. The chances of success are lower than with systematic therapy designed and supervised by professionals.

Self-help groups

Although people who stutter come in all shapes and sizes, not many of them like working in groups. The effort of speaking is too great. Consequently stutterers' self-help groups are slow to get started, and many simply fade away.

Even the successful and progressive groups have remarkably few members considering the number of people afflicted by stuttering. The National Stuttering Project in the United States,[6] for example, is well established and active. It is efficiently run by full-time staff, but its membership of 1,500 is only about 0.06 per cent of the stuttering population. The situation in Canada is similar. Lack of funds is partly responsible for this, but the people who stutter are also responsible. They are reluctant to come out into the open and say, 'Here we are! We are ordinary people, but we can't speak very well. We'd just like a little help and understanding.'

I have tremendous admiration for a small self-help group of spastics in Victoria, British Columbia. The members have great difficulty speaking clearly and have problems with their muscle control, but they travel from church to church standing up and telling people about themselves. Without self-pity they try to show that behind the distressing physical and vocal facades there are warm, loving human beings with much to offer the world if society will let them. They don't ask a normal person to speak for them. They don't plead. They just describe the facts. It takes a great deal of courage.

If more stutterers would come out of their closets, join such groups, and learn to bear or even fight rejection, ridicule, and discrimination in good company, they would find the pain far less than the anguish of fear and self-inflicted loneliness.

The self-help organizations have numerous active chapters in the United States, Canada, Britain, Sweden, Germany, and Australia, but these groups can help only if the stutterers will contribute and participate. Some of the groups just provide a place where people who stutter can get together and talk without the ridicule and censure of society. It helps to know you are not alone. The relief of being able to talk openly about stuttering and the problems it causes can be tremendous.

Some groups take a somewhat militant stance. The P-club in Sweden for example, has taken action against inaccurate, damaging statements in the media about people who stutter. This group seems to be changing public opinion. Other groups are tied to a particular type of speech therapy or even to a particular hospital and provide ex-patients with a critical audience that helps them keep their speech techniques in line.

Anybody wanting help can contact these groups. A few addresses are listed in appendices. Talking with the members will give a good idea of where the best therapy can be found.

Speech therapists and patients: the informal contract

When a therapist accepts a stuttering patient for treatment there is an unspoken and unwritten contract. The therapist agrees to use her skills, and the stutterer agrees to work hard and persevere. Guiding a person with a severe stutter to better fluency is often painful and frustrating for both the therapist and the patient. The therapists invest a tremendous amount of themselves in their patients, particularly when they use stuttering modification therapy to treat the stutterer as a whole person. If the treatment fails, no matter how professional and objective the therapist is, there are likely to be feelings of guilt on both sides that need to be resolved. The therapist walks a razor's edge of emotional involvement. She must remain friendly with the patients without forming close friendships that would detract from the treatment. Speech therapy can be a very intimate and emotional business, and efforts need to be made by both therapists and patients to avoid the formation of bonds that are too close for comfort.

I was involved in an intensive course of speech therapy using innovative approaches that made great demands on the trust, courage, and emotions of the patients. We all felt shattered by the end of the second week, but most of us were much more fluent. A rising tide of emotional involvement was dealt with gently but firmly by the therapists, who were well aware of the tensions and ties that can develop between people sharing stress, fear, and pain.

Speech pathologists bring a degree of concerned professionalism to their work that has earned my unqualified respect.

What happens when speech therapy succeeds?

Adult stutterers like to daydream about what life would be like without a stutter. I could never understand what stopped anybody with normal speech from becoming Prime Minister, or at least a member of the Cabinet. Aiming a little lower, a person afflicted with a stutter may well think how pleasant it would be to be able to hold forth at committee meetings, ask questions at conferences, fluently court a pretty girl, and burn the ears of impudent telephone operators. He thinks of all the social situations he avoids because of the effort and embarrassment of having to talk and the signs of rejection on the faces of people he meets. He could get a date with the brunette he met on the ski slopes if only he could say all the right words without blocking. He could learn another language just for fun. He sees new vistas opening before him and may feel there would be nothing he couldn't do and nothing to fear if he were fluent.

The changes improved fluency make in a stutterer's life depend upon the person. If he is fundamentally a blockhead, he'll just become a blockhead without a stutter. If he's a genius, he'll still be a genius, but better able to tell people about it rather than hide his light under a bushel of uncontrolled repetitions and hesitations. A person with a slight stutter who achieves almost complete fluency will just be less nervous about the possibility that his speech will let him down. Someone who has had a severe, debilitating stutter for a long time may react profoundly to improved fluency. It depends upon how far the handicap has initially affected a person's life style and over-all social behaviour.

Most people who stutter severely delude themselves that their antipathy to the telephone, public speaking, large parties, committee meetings, and appearing on radio or television is wholly the result of their stuttering. They ignore the fact that many people with normal speech are terrified of the telephone, speaking in public, parties, and radio and television appearances. The improved fluency may or may not reduce a stutterer's hang-ups about situations he finds difficult. He may be so programmed to associate telephones with dislike that he cannot change.

All handicapped people who resolve their disability to the extent that it is no longer an appreciable handicap must deal with society's new perception of them and with their own changed perceptions of their surroundings. Recovery from a severe disorder can be a mixed blessing.

A freckled, red-haired boy, aged about seven, had been completely deaf and almost mute all his life until he had an operation that gave him normal hearing. I met him about a month after his surgery, when he was learning to speak. He was nervous and jumpy. When I spoke to him his eyes widened with fear, and it was clear that he didn't entirely understand what I said. This was to be expected in view of my partial disfluency and his previous deafness, but I was puzzled by his obvious fear until his mother explained.

The boy had never heard anybody speak, hammer in a nail, laugh, or sneeze, and the noise of the traffic, the wail of ambulance sirens, and the music on the radio were completely unfamiliar to him. He didn't yet associate speech with communication, music with pleasure, or sounds with activities and objects. I get jumpy at our cottage in the bush when I hear an unfamiliar noise in the middle of the night. Is it a raccoon, or a bear, or an intruder? The small boy had just encountered a host of unfamiliar sounds full of the menace of the unknown. He was sorting them out and learning to live in his new and noisy world. I was told he overcame this perceptual problem in a few months, his fears giving way to excitement.

A more extreme and tragic example of the difficulties a person with severely impaired perception experiences when adapting to newly restored faculties is the well-documented case of S.B., the fifty-two-year-old Englishman who lost his sight as a child and had it restored in 1958 by a brilliant eye operation. His response to being able to see was observed by the British psychiatrist Richard Gregory, who described the case in 'Recovery from early blindness: a case study.'[7] Richard Restak has also discussed S.B.'s case, in the context of perception of reality by man and other mammals, in his excellent and thought-provoking book *The Brain: The Last Frontier*.[8]

S.B. could see quite well, but had difficulty perceiving height and recognizing objects by their visible shapes. His drawings of objects left out important features, but he learned to associate things he knew from their feel when he was blind with what he saw with his eyes. Before he regained his sight he was a cheerful, confident, dominant man, who coped with heavy traffic and earned a good living repairing shoes. He was well adapted to his sightless life and enjoyed what he perceived by touch, smell, and hearing.

Soon after he regained his sight he began to deteriorate mentally and became a recluse, sitting in the dark for long periods. He found the visible world a drab place. His attempts to pull himself out of his downward slide failed. Everything disappointed him, and gradually he lost his peace of mind and self-respect.

When he was blind, every time he overcame his handicap it was an achievement, and the psychiatrist felt that, when S.B. could see, these triumphs seemed insignificant. S.B. became deeply depressed and died in 1960, less than two years after his eye operation. This is an extreme and sad case, but it illustrates the dangers of rehabilitating a person with a perceptual handicap if he is well adapted to his disability.

Recovery can be a mixed blessing, and it is unwise for a person who stutters to have false expectations about what life will be like when he becomes more fluent. He may be disappointed and find that some of the barriers between himself and society that he assumed were caused by his stuttering remain when he speaks more easily. A boy at my preparatory school, who threw up every time he became nervous, had a bad time with his peers and acquired the unenviable nickname of Spewky Sidney or S.S. He overcame his nausea, but still had a bad time because his large ears stuck out and he lisped. He kept his nickname. Blackbirds peck at birds of any other colour, not only white, and it doesn't always help to moult and grow more orthodox feathers.

I am not aware of any case history of the effects on the life of an adult with a severe, self-reinforcing stutter when he achieved a high degree of fluency. I know about mild stutterers who became very fluent and entered new and more challenging jobs. Some of these fluent stutterers enhanced their careers at the price of disrupting their families, but there could have been reasons other than the new fluency.

My own case is not clear-cut because I still stutter, but my speech control and social relationships have greatly improved in the last twenty years. My stutter was very severe and affected both my daily communication and my health. Now that I speak more easily and have arranged my life so that I speak less, my health has improved. This is, of course, welcome. The telephone is no longer a nightmare, and I use it frequently, which saves time. My temper has a longer fuse now that I can express my displeasure. I can interview and be interviewed more freely, and I don't avoid public exposure. People say that I am more outgoing, and I am conscious of being more relaxed about life. I no longer need to fight for survival every day.

All these can be listed on the credit side of the ledger. The debit side contains one item that I share with the unfortunate S.B. When I was very inarticulate, any successful communication was a major achievement, and overcoming almost insurmountable obstacles gave me daily kicks. Even such a small speech success as ordering breakfast in a restaurant was deeply satisfying. I miss the daily sense of achievement and have taken on new challenges – one of which is writing this book.

Some people who stutter develop acute senses and an exceptional ability to receive and send the unspoken part of communication. I was afraid that I would lose this if I became more fluent, but if anything these senses have sharpened now that speech is a larger part of my communicative amalgam. My case is very different from S.B.'s. He was completely adapted to his blindness and enjoyed his other senses. I coped with my stuttering and adapted in many ways, but no person who stutters severely fully adapts to the rejections of society.

As speech therapy improves and we learn more about the

cerebral processes involved in speech and emotion, people with severe stutters may become much more fluent with less effort. When this happens it may be necessary for therapists to extend their mandate so as to help recently fluent patients deal with their new perceptions, roles, and relationships with society.

SEVEN

The odyssey to fluent stuttering

'... a journey into the future, a hunting after happiness.'

William Stakhel

There is a wide gap between reading about stuttering theory and the reality of intensive treatment. If I had known what was ahead when I decided to have intensive speech therapy I doubt that I'd have had the courage to start the long journey to fluent stuttering. When I walked the high mountains in winter and fought fatigue, wind, and bitter cold, I often exclaimed, 'What the hell am I doing here?' During the more demanding parts of speech therapy, I said the same thing many times.

All my previous treatments had been fairly brief – about six months or less – and were carried out in the cosy, supportive confines of the clinics. I was not aware that my new treatment would persist for several years. Moreover, although I knew that situational and group therapies were involved, I had no real idea what they meant. Unwittingly, I was embarking on an odyssey in a leaky cockleshell of a boat of stuttering theory accompanied by a crew I didn't know. The skipper, to my dismay, would hand over the boat to the bewildered crew as soon as we were out of harbour so she could concentrate on therapeutic navigation.

The word 'situation' didn't bother me, but the thought of group therapy certainly did. It appalled me. Not being a groupie, I preferred to work and play with a few companions and was reluctant to involve myself with masses of humanity.

I felt that all medical treatment should be a private affair and was never especially keen on being a patient in those teaching hospitals where they bring students to view the ailing bodies while nurses flourish enema tubes in the background. Proposing that I should cold-bloodedly expose my speech – and my feelings about it – to a large group of strangers was like asking me to go to a nudist colony where the world would see all my moles, warts, and goose bumps. My first reaction was, 'Group therapy? Forget it!'

It turned out that the group work was the most enjoyable part of the therapy, and I made many lasting friends. It was the situational therapy that gave all of us the most trouble. It is all very well to expose your articulatory weaknesses to other people with stutters in the clinic, but taking these weaknesses out onto the street or displaying them on national television at prime time takes a great deal of *chutzpah*. This Yiddish word, which means shameless audacity, best describes what is demanded of patients in situational therapy. They need the audacity to approach strangers and stutter openly, deliberately, and fluently without feeling ashamed of their way of speaking. Without *chutzpah* the stutterer is lost.

During my preliminary assessment at the Royal Ottawa Hospital, the attractive speech therapist was coolly efficient, but when I unfolded my history of unsuccessful treatment a wary look came into her eye. Consider her position. Here was I, a talkative, stuttering scientist who had responded poorly to forty years or more of treatment and who clearly had reservations about speech therapy and even about speech therapists in general. It might be that I was an unusually resistant patient who couldn't or wouldn't co-operate; or it might be that I'd just had the wrong kind of treatment. What were the chances of even partial success? Obviously the prognosis was not good. No wonder she looked wary. Should she invest her time and the government's money in a lost cause? Much later she confessed that she was not at all keen to take me on.

She passed me to another attractive woman clinician, a psychometrist – the type of psychologist who measures the relative strength of your mind. My past experience of psychologists and other types of mind-benders had been mixed, and my feelings were ambivalent. I wasn't keen on

another Freudian probe into the murkier corners of my
libido, so I was cautious and parried some of the preliminary
questions with a nimble riposte or two learned on past
therapeutic battlefields. I relaxed when the conversation
didn't stray below my chin, and it became apparent that this
particular clinician was taking a refreshingly empirical,
behavioural approach rather than asking me to wade ankle
deep in the suppositions of a Freudian quagmire. Best of all,
she had a puckish sense of humour and a fine nose for the
ridiculous, so I knew we would get along as sparring partners.
Unknown to me, she didn't share my enthusiasm, and she ad-
mitted later that she was shattered by the thought of having
me as a patient. She went home and cried.

I nearly flunked my assessment. I thought I'd behaved
myself remarkably well during the cross-examinations. I
hadn't let on that I knew a little about the etiology and treatment of stuttering, because no clinician likes a smart aleck for
a client. I politely shut up and let the therapists have their say
and regarded myself as the perfect potential patient. The
therapists' collective misgivings puzzled me.

Maybe it was the challenge or possibly just plain compassion, but they let me reach first base and try a few preliminary
sessions. After they realized that I was co-operative, we all
got along famously during the several years of treatment. All
the therapists at the ROH's Speech Rehabilitation Unit (now
Communication Disorders) were, and still are as far as I
know, highly efficient and dedicated young women. The fact
that they were also lively, intelligent, and attractive did not
detract in the least from the therapy.

The early part of the treatment was on a one-to-one basis.
At first the clinician tested my vocal capabilities and designed
a plan of attack. My stuttering wasn't causing me too many
problems in my daily life, although I found talking all the
time in my job exceedingly tiring. Stress was building up, but
in retrospect it was probably largely caused by the frustration
of working for a bureaucracy. I had some difficulty reducing
my rate of speaking, prolonging words, and using voluntary
repetition in the early therapy sessions and was strongly conditioned to stutter in response to many word and situation
cues – even in my sleep. I also had a deeply ingrained anxiety

about stuttering and was tense before and during speaking. In retrospect, I was a prime candidate for integrated therapy consisting of both stuttering modification and fluency shaping.

It turned out that I received therapy to reduce anxiety, modify my attitudes, learn to prolong sounds and words, practise easy onset to beginnings of words, develop smooth verbal continuity using voluntary controlled repetition (VCR), reduce my rate of speaking, learn to relax before and during speech, respond better to stuttering cues, and increase my tolerance to speech frustration. Desensitization, group discussion, and exercises for transferring the new speech techniques to real situations with all their tensions were also included. These methods contain elements of the treatments designed by Bryng Bryngelson, Wendell Johnson, Joseph G. Sheehan, Charles Van Riper, and Webster, together with a spot of psychotherapeutic counselling. A novel element in the therapy was that as soon as a patient improved he was permitted to monitor other stutterers until, finally, when he had much better control, he graduated to Hospital Volunteer (with free parking privileges) and helped himself by helping others. This could be regarded as a form of operant conditioning, the Hospital Volunteer status being the reward, but there was little evidence of penalties. Whatever the basis, for many patients it was a highly effective treatment.

The therapy involved practice, practice, practice. There are many examples of patients who received therapy and later became speech therapists themselves so they could maintain their fluency by constant exposure to the speech techniques they taught. It is quite believable, because the best results come from constant practice.

The therapy was complex, but it was carried out in such a skilful, orderly way that there was no confusion. Each component of the treatment supplemented the others at the right stages and the emphasis of each phase could be shifted to suit the needs of individuals. It was a flexible, many-pronged approach on a wide front.

For a few weeks, the therapy was low key and consisted of designing graduated daily exercises, starting with short sentences and progressing to stages of increasing difficulty. I taped my disfluency and listened to my new speech, which soon became – at least in the clinic – a smooth flow like a meandering river instead of my usual verbal rapids, eddies, and whirlpools. I was gradually exposed to speaking situations in the hospital that involved talking to staff and patients. Success varied, but I developed a lot more nerve and learned a great deal about people.

The nerve developed because I was asked to go into the busy hospital dining room, select someone at random, introduce myself and say, 'May I sit here? I am receiving speech therapy and would like to practise my speaking techniques.' This took a great deal of guts – more than I thought I had. You never knew what kind of person you would get. Some were welcoming and co-operative, others said, 'Yes, I do mind! Get lost!' A panicky few fled to the washroom; some valiantly stuck it out but were clearly embarrassed; and one woman ignored me completely. Once I sat with a young psychiatric patient who was friendly and chatty but emphasized his philosophical points by stabbing the table violently with his fork until it bent, just inches from my chest.

There are some people who can walk up to strangers and start chatting. I am not one of them. I was so conditioned by my stoic British education, where it was 'just not done' and a 'poor show' to thrust yourself upon a stranger, that I had to make an enormous effort just to say 'Good morning' to a passer-by. It was not shyness, just custom. All these social inhibitions were cast to the winds during the first few weeks of therapy as I learned to chat to perfect strangers at the drop of a hat, stutter and all.

During this phase I visited the hidden side of society's moon, the world of the handicapped. Everybody knows the disabled are there, but most people prefer them out of sight and out of mind. At that time the Royal Ottawa Hospital Speech Rehabilitation Unit was housed in the same complex as other units for helping people severely handicapped by automobile accidents and strokes to cope with their disabilities. The situational speech exercises allowed me to meet young people who, with no hint of self-pity, cheerfully faced the consequences of terrible injuries, and older people, partly paralysed and nearly speechless from cerebral thromboses and aneurisms, who faced their limited futures with courage and dignity. It was a heart-rending yet heart-warming experience. It would be salutary for people who drink and drive to be compelled, as part of their sentences, to visit or even assist patients in the rehabilitation wards, where physiotherapists work so hard to help accident victims with spinal or cerebral injuries to lead more normal lives.

With a great deal of effort I was able to speak to many individuals in the hospital using the new methods. The speaking situations were carefully graded until I was able to talk to audiences of several people. The supportive atmosphere of the clinic improved my speech considerably within a few weeks, the only real remaining bugbear being the telephone.

Nobody can imagine the difficulties a person with a stutter has on the telephone unless they stutter themselves. Direct dialling has, of course, been a help. Before it was introduced it was exceedingly difficult for a stutterer to reel off long numbers to impatient operators. For many the telephone was not a viable means of communication. Even with direct dialling it is sometimes necessary to give a credit-card number for a long-distance call, and this is nearly impossible for a person with a severe stutter. At some stage you have to say who you are and what you want. There is no escaping the fact that the purpose of the telephone is to speak to somebody.

The first spoken words on the telephone at the clinic were voluntarily repeated in a slow, prolonged manner to signal the listener that the speaker had a speech impediment and no doubt about it. If a person with a stutter tries to hide his disability, the listener gets nervous and may think the speaker is drunk or making a silent, heavy-breathing, obscene phone call. Hundreds of times people on the telephone have said to me, 'There seems to be something wrong with the line,' when nonplussed by my silent blocks. My usual reply is, 'The line's okay. I have a stutter,' which I can usually say quite fluently.

Once a person knows you stutter, there's a fair chance of a reasonable response, but not always. The preliminaries were always the hard part, and it took tremendous concentration to speak and voluntarily repeat words and sounds fluently instead of blocking. Thereafter it was necessary to keep the rate of speaking down below sixty words a minute, to approach words gently and smoothly, and to keep up the flow during the dialogue.

The early telephone calls within the hospital were not too difficult, but when calls were made outside the clinic, most patients, including myself, had a great deal of trouble. As far as possible I made real-life outside calls to my bank, hotel, or office, but sometimes I faked it and tried calls to restaurants, hotels, car-hire firms, bus terminals, travel agents, and airline offices. The airlines were the best, because they usually replied with a recorded message saying they were busy and would the caller please call back – it enabled me honourably to cop out of an assignment that produced a cold sweat.

Hotels and restaurants varied in their difficulty. The telephone operators in the large, expensive hotels are trained to be polite and cope dispassionately with fires, earthquakes, cranks, and people struggling with a stutter. Calling was easy. I awarded the first prize for difficulty to telephone operators in small motels in Hull, across the river from Ottawa. They were usually so rude when you stuttered that they were a marvellous challenge. Fortunately they couldn't see my digital gestures (body language?) while I calmly and politely persisted with my questions, using voluntary repetition of sounds and prolonging the words. Busy bus companies were tough to deal with; they were impatient rather than rude, and I appreciated their reasons for being so. Salesmen wanting to sell you something, as at the car-hire firms, were pushovers. They'd have been polite if you'd asked the cost of hiring a Cadillac for a month in disfluent Kurdish.

These assignments provided insights into the ways different sectors of society respond to a stutter, even a controlled stutter, with its prolonged words and repeated sounds. In general, people who were under great stress or who belonged to ethnic groups that normally speak very quickly (e.g., Italian, French, and Spanish) responded badly to disfluency, which is understandable. I learned to arrange my unwitting telephone audiences into carefully graded degrees of difficulty.

Succeeding with the telephone can be quite a shock. A sixty-year-old executive had never been able to call his wife on the telephone because of his severe blocks. During a carefully controlled phone assignment he spoke fluently to her for about ten minutes, put down the telephone, and unashamedly wept.

Gradually the components of the therapy began to fall into place. It was like learning to drive a car. At first there were too many things to remember. It was vital that each step was carried out in the right sequence or the speech engine stalled. After a great deal of practice everything became more or less automatic, but you couldn't afford to relax your vigilance. If you did so you sooner or later collided with a difficult word and blocked your verbal traffic.

About this time I developed what I called the Stutterer's Credo as an *aide mémoire*.

The Stutterer's Credo

I believe that I can maintain fluent speech provided that:
I *prolong* my words and *speak slowly* at a rate I can manage;
I use *voluntary controlled repetition* to signal people that
  I stutter and to help me past potential blocks;
I approach the beginnings of words *gently* and slowly;
I *never push past blocks*;
I *pause (i.e., cancel) when I block*, and try again,
  approaching the word slowly and smoothly, using
  voluntary controlled repetition when necessary;
I *never* try to avoid a block by *substituting* an easy
  word for a hard word;
I *remain in contact* with the audience and myself, and keep
  sufficient eye contact not to cause embarrassment;
I *never avoid a speaking situation* just because I
  stutter (within the limits of common sense);
I *never hide my stutter* from myself or other people;
I *practise* good speech technique as often as possible
  in order to stutter in a fluent manner that will
  not interrupt communication.

I added another private component later: 'I shall *never* lose my temper with people who react rudely to my stuttering but, for the sake of other stutterers, I must *never* let them get away with it.'

The voluntary controlled repetition is the hardest part for me to maintain. Van Riper's cancellation of blocks is in the credo, and so is avoiding avoidance, which both work when I remember them. The gentle approach (easy onset) to words has echoes of fluency shaping therapy, and the attitude components reflect the psychotherapeutic aspects of speech modification therapy.

Over the years the therapy has continued to evolve and is still changing. In recent years therapists have placed much greater emphasis on the type of fluency shaping described by Webster,[1] but this varies from one clinic to another.

I used the Stutterer's Credo as my guiding light for several years. I still use it to refresh my memory about what I should be doing when I stray away from the path of vocal righteousness, which I do all too frequently.

If Moses could have included the credo in his famous tablets, maybe his stuttering would have improved. In any case he had an excellent therapist: 'And Moses said unto the Lord, "O my Lord I am not eloquent ... but I am slow of speech, and of a slow tongue." ... And the Lord said unto him ... "I will be with thy mouth ... and will teach you what ye shall do." '

Moses did something that makes most therapists shudder. He let his brother Aaron speak for him (Exodus 4:10–15; 27–30). He *avoided*.

Once I had grasped the basics, I soon became remarkably fluent within the hospital and was ready for greater challenges. When I was introduced to the main group it needed a major effort to overcome my antipathy to talking to large audiences. My speech became incredibly brittle and kept collapsing without warning, because the new and larger audience seemed to prevent me from using the speech techniques I had learned. The problem of audience interaction reared its head and became the heart of future difficulties.

I knew that when I used the new speech techniques I could stutter fluently in a manner that did not disrupt communication, but in difficult situations something prevented me from using the techniques. It was like being given a key to a locked chest full of my most precious possessions that only opened the lock when I was on my own and jammed when I wanted to open the chest to show the contents to other people. The precious possessions were the multitude of things I wanted to say. On my own I could say them, but could not always do so with other people present.

I chipped away for months at the solid wall that prevented me from using the wonderful new way of speaking. Eventually, the barrier disappeared, but even today it tends to return without warning and makes it difficult for me to use the techniques. In the most difficult situations I use the Edinburgh Masker. Although some therapists look upon it as a cop-out, or distraction, or a form of avoidance, I feel it is common sense to use it when the likelihood of speech failure is very high.

The speech therapist and psychometrist worked valiantly to remove this *something* – the wall that stopped me using the techniques. It would have helped if we had known what the something was! It was clear to me that this was the factor that had prevented me from responding to earlier therapy. Speculating, it seems likely that the wall was built during the many years of associating certain circumstances with stuttering and was constructed from a multitude of conditioned responses to difficult speaking situations. This subliminal conditioning is very hard to break, and the wall was a tangible, frustrating reality, an almost impermeable block to progress.

The power of the mental block is illustrated by what happened to me on one outside speech assignment in a shopping plaza. I went from store to store trying to use prolongation, repetition, and slow speech. Without warning my mind blanked out the well-learned methods for about fifteen minutes. I couldn't remember anything about the Stutterer's Credo or my therapist's guidelines. It took some time to get back in gear.

With months of practice and gradual desensitization, the wall began to crumble. My diary at that time says 'I tell myself to prolong and repeat, but sometimes nothing happens. I have been given a key that doesn't quite fit the lock. Chipping at this wall week after week has made some dents in its face, but the wall tends to return. Each time, however, the chips get larger and the wall gradually crumbles, leaving debris on the ground. At first I tripped over the pieces when I was careless or tired, but now I can chart my way around the remaining obstacles without too much trouble.'

This was one of the hardest tasks I have ever undertaken, and it made great demands upon my inner resources. Without the help of the therapists and the support of my companions in the group I don't think I could have persevered. By no means all stutterers have these barriers to using the prescribed speaking techniques, and some, particularly the younger people, seem able to use them quite freely.

A small group of about ten selected patients underwent concentrated therapy for ten hours or more every week-day for two weeks. Some sessions lasted until 11 PM, and by the end of the course both the therapists and the patients were visibly wilting. Every day started with simple word and sentence exercises to reinforce the prolongation and voluntary controlled repetition techniques and get the feel of different rates of speaking (40, 60, 80, or 100 words per minute) using stop-watches and tape recorders. Each day there were sessions on closed-circuit television, but in the afternoons we went in pairs to the shopping plazas, restaurants, and government offices to try out the techniques. Evenings were spent in group sessions discussing the philosophy of the therapy and refining the method. The grand finale was the challenge of a ten-minute presentation in front of an audience of thirty people. At the end of the two weeks we were all much more fluent in the clinic and had better carry-over in the outside world. We had taken a big step, but still had a long way to go.

It is worth giving more details about one or two points that came up during the course. My block about using the techniques was tackled intensively with desensitization sessions. I had many stuttering cues to contend with, but we managed to focus on a few of the main ones, which included taxis, hotels, lecture theatres, crowds, and, of course, the telephone. For hours on end, I was shown colour slide after colour slide illustrating these situations and I had to talk about each of them. At first my mental block inhibited the use of speech techniques, but gradually, when I was nearly exhausted and my eyes burned from looking at the slides, I found that I was using the speech techniques much more freely. This did carry over to the outside world.

My problem with the stuttering cues presented by telephones and lecture theatres still persists to a lesser degree, but ever since this therapy I have had little or no trouble with taxis, hotels, and other situations covered during these tiring sessions. My inhibiting blocks had dissolved in the solvent of pure boredom during the slide sessions. It was, of course, a form of conditioning, but it seemed to be the only quick way to dissipate the effects of inhibiting cues. It was very hard on the clinician.

The television sessions were terrifying at first, but they were invaluable once we became used to the gadgetry. The patient was videotaped while reading aloud or discussing his speech with the therapist; later he saw the playback. The first and last tapes were useful demonstrations of the change in our speech during the treatment. Most of all, however, the TV sessions forced the patient to accept the reality of his stutter, to scrutinize his speech in great detail, and to recognize bad habits. At first the replays in front of the group were embarrassing, but we soon learned to trust each other and to become more objective.

The videotapes brought us down to earth with a bump. I was horrified that my face looked like that of a stranger much less interesting than myself. I stuttered in minor ways (quite apart from the major blocks) much more than I had realized – I was so used to the lesser disfluencies and so adept at self-deception that they did not register. My nose, bashed about in past rugby encounters, looked like a crooked lump, and the resonant voice I thought I heard every day came over as a plummy English accent. I was disillusioned with my television image and, on the first replay, cried, 'Is that me? Oh, my God!'

When I stuttered on the screen, I didn't like it at all. It hardened my resolve to change my speech behaviour. When I went over the tapes I could compare what I did when I was fluent with what happened when I blocked. Gradually, I modified my speech behaviour. We all found it a challenge to meet our true selves, accept our stutters, and do something about it. At the end of the session I was interviewed by another stutterer for twenty minutes about photography during World War II. By using the speaking techniques, we managed to give a virtually flawless performance.

A few of us were selected to carry this television work over into the all-too-real world in a way that would terrify anybody. A national television network wanted some of us to show the public how the therapy was carried out and how the techniques were used outside the clinic. I was selected for the situation exercise.

I set up a session in a florist's shop and self-consciously walked into the store and asked a girl about how to look after plants while cameras, mikes, and lights hovered around. Although I was jittery, I used voluntary controlled repetition, cancellation, and prolongation without too much difficulty. The session ended, and I thankfully wiped the sweat from my brow and walked outside. To my horror I was interviewed again in front of a large crowd of curious onlookers attracted by all the paraphernalia of the media. I felt sick, but managed to maintain the speech techniques for a remarkably long ten minutes until it was all over. In retrospect, it went very well. The stress wasn't caused by stage fright, but by the effort of maintaining the speech techniques in such a challenging situation. I hoped they'd cut my clip from the television program, but I had no such luck. I appeared three times on the news at prime time and groaned every time I saw it.

The evening after this television trauma I went shopping in a large plaza on the other side of town. To my surprise, several strangers came up and congratulated me on the performance. Best of all, some of them said, 'I never understood what was involved in a stutter and how hard it is to treat. Where can we find out more about it?' It was worth every shattered nerve.

Most patients were nervous about testing the speech techniques in public, because failures were embarrassing. But when the techniques did succeed it was amazing how store clerks responded to controlled, prolonged, deliberately repetitive speech instead of an uncontrolled series of stumbles and blocks. As long as continuous communication was maintained, even with an unusual amount of repetition, the disfluency didn't matter. The audiences did not become tense and difficult, and the better feedback helped the stutterers' speech. The therapists had told us that people responded better to controlled disfluency than uncontrolled stuttering, but not all of us believed them. Nevertheless they were right.

The clinicians put us through these difficult therapeutic hoops, so it was only fitting that they should show us how to do it. I greatly admired their courage when, although they had normal speech, they went into stores and acted as though they had, first, uncontrolled stutters, and then controlled disfluency, so that we could see the differences in feedback. As the therapists struggled not to appear embarrassed they came in for a great deal of good-natured ribbing from the patients.

These public speech exercises were sometimes funny. One class was at the stage of deliberately repeating the first sounds of nearly every word all through the day. A group of them stood talking like slow machine-guns on a crowded escalator in a shopping plaza. A stout man just ahead heard this extraordinary chatter and turned around to stare as the steps bore him downwards. He was so fascinated that he forgot to step off the escalator and fell on his bottom at the end with all the other people piling on top of him in sheer pandemonium.

A tall burly farmer was asked by the therapist to go to busy Elgin Street in Ottawa and ask people the time, or directions to stores or restaurants, using his new techniques, just for practice. He accosted several people and was doing remarkably well until he saw across the street a scruffy-looking individual bumming quarters from passers-by. He was making angry gestures and clearly objected to the farmer trespassing on his territory. The large stutterer crossed the street and, looming over the vagrant, said in a low conspiratorial voice with perfectly controlled deliberate repetition, 'You bum this side, bud, and I'll bum the other.'

My most expensive situational-therapy experience occurred when I went into an art shop to try out my controlled repetition. It worked all too well. I walked out clutching a $250 painting of a winter scene.

After the intensive course of therapy, most of us had much better speech, but in the following weeks the benefit tended to fade under the pressures of the outside world. The real work of maintaining the speech began.

It was a long, slow slog and involved doing speech exercises for many hours a day at home, with regular visits to the clinic to reinforce the technique when it became sloppy. Some of the patients relapsed, others went on to much better speech, and most of us fought to hold onto our gains. The better speech increased confidence and reduced stress, and the truth of Van Riper's theory that *felt fluency* helps the stutterer became apparent. Before therapy, a stutterer's speech would plunge into an uncontrollable downward spiral to inarticulacy, the poor speech making the speech worse. After therapy, many of us could control the spiral and avoid the previous severe regressions that could last for several weeks.

After therapy, any adult who has stuttered severely for many years needs to be continually vigilant. When his speech regresses, he gets out his tape recorder, listens to what he is doing wrong, and practises the correct methods. Some stutters disappear almost completely, but not many adults have that much luck.

Some of us have been on refresher mini-courses to keep us on track. During these courses, it was obvious that speech therapy is evolving, with more emphasis on easy, gentle approaches to words, slower speech, and prolongation, and less concern with voluntary stuttering. The methods used by the different clinics vary. In the best of them, the approach is innovative, experimental, and empirical. The stuttering syndrome is so complex that we still have a long way to go before therapy can be placed on a firm scientific basis.

People who have been on these intensive courses develop a tremendous respect for the therapists. The clinicians operate within definite therapeutic guidelines, but need to be sensitive to a stutterer's needs and to use their intuition to forecast how the patient will respond to certain patterns of treatment. Some therapists seem to know what is going on inside a stutterer's head and to be able to predict his fears, but treatment sessions can be exhausting and frustrating. Genuine, qualified therapists (not the quacks) undergo rigorous training, require great skill, and work incredibly hard.

EIGHT

Living with an albatross around your neck: stutterers and society

'A man cannot be measured by the colour of his skin, or by his speech, or by his clothes or jewels, but only by his heart.'

Mika Waltari

A few years ago there was a story going around spastic circles in Canada about a severely disabled young man who was taken in his wheelchair to a shopping plaza. His disability was obvious: he had great difficulty controlling the movement of his limbs; his head tended to loll to one side; and when he tried to speak, his face contorted and the sounds that emerged were hard to understand. As his chair was wheeled past the stores, he was suddenly confronted by a burly, red-faced man who angrily shouted, 'Why do you filthy, ugly people come here? Stay away! Stay in the institution where nobody can see you.'

Many handicapped people encounter rejections that are not quite so traumatic, but if their handicap is obvious people tend to avoid them and occasionally react violently. A young man in Victoria, British Columbia, who is a spastic, was beaten up by louts as he walked home from therapy with a friend, simply because he walked and talked in a strange way. I learned as a young man to be wary when I spoke in certain bars because my stuttering attracted attention and sometimes triggered a fracas. It is the old story about society's reaction to someone who is different. The more obvious the difference, the greater the reaction.

A person with a mild stutter may have a few social problems, and at one time it was even fashionable to stutter – wealthy aristocrats in Britain cultivated a vague, stuttering, stumbling way of speaking as a mark of their status. Nevertheless, a person with a very severe stutter who grimaces, twitches, and contorts his face in his efforts to speak is likely to encounter social difficulties.

A young woman in a wheelchair who found it difficult to set up house with other handicapped people in an Ottawa suburb because of local residents' objections, said on television that 'Canadians just don't like the handicapped.' It is not only Canadians who react adversely to the disabled, and it is not just a case of liking or disliking. In this case, the residents were probably afraid that a colony of handicapped people would reduce real-estate values; but usually the reasons for such behaviour are more complex. It is easy to apply such words as 'insensitive,' 'selfish,' and 'cruel,' but unreasoning fear of the unfamiliar, the unknown, and the uncontrolled runs through people's behaviour toward the handicapped. There is some truth in the old English proverb that cruelty is a tyrant that is always attended by fear. Those who respond well to the handicapped are able to override their fears by intelligence, humanity, compassion, and a felt need to probe beneath the surface and understand.

Some sociologists say that society's response to the handicapped is a reflection of the inbuilt attribute of animal populations to reject or attack any individual who looks, acts, or smells different from the norm. However, man has a well-developed brain. He is more than just an animal responding unthinkingly to fear and uncertainty. We may have inherited a rag-bag of nasty behavioural traits, but our large convoluted, cerebral cortex enables us to monitor and modify these urges. If it didn't, no nubile female would be safe on the street. Man is not just the slave of inherited behaviour. Society may have inbuilt responses to the handicapped, but individuals possess brains that permit choices of behaviour.

A wealthy woman, one of the Beautiful People, once said to me, 'I try to be kind to handicapped people I meet, but *really* ... ! I just can't stand to see them. I simply tell them to go away. What else can I do?' She responded to her feelings of revulsion and fear without any visible signs of other cerebral activity. She had the choice of rejecting the handicapped or of making an effort to look beyond the surface and establish contact. She chose the easier course. I reminded her that I was a handicapped person with a severe speech defect. She looked startled and retorted, 'You're different. I've known you since you were a child,' and thereby put her finger on the problem of her relationship with the disabled. It was her fear of the unfamiliar and unpredictable that disturbed her, not just the disability.

Some people may argue that severe stuttering, with its on-and-off occurrence, cannot be regarded as a disability in the same way as the physical handicaps of paraplegics, the deaf, and the blind; but very severe stuttering can be as disabling as many major problems of limb control, hearing, and even sight. I was once asked, 'If you had the choice of having a severe, debilitating stutter or being blind, which would you take?' The question seemed an easy one to answer, but it took me several minutes to think about it. My reply was that I'd rather be blind, because society to some extent accepts blind people and allows for their disability. Sightless people, although they miss a great deal, can communicate effectively and participate in society in many ways. A person who stutters very severely is denied effective communication most of the time, and the attitudes of society limit his social activities unless he is very determined indeed. He can all too easily be forced to live in the dark, lonely cave of his own mind.

Adverse responses to stuttering often arise because most people do not appreciate the difficulties a person with a stutter encounters in the ordinary, daily communication that fluent speakers take for granted. Most people have no idea of the stutterer's hidden, everyday world.

The paradox

People in Western societies live in an age of enlightenment. Social services help the aged, the sick, the poor, and the disadvantaged. Research is funded by governments – sometimes grudgingly – to find ways of reducing the physical and mental woes of mankind. The brutality of nineteenth-century society toward many of its members seems mere history: mentally handicapped people are no longer chained in the squalor of Bedlam; eccentric women aren't burned as witches; and crippled people no longer need to beg – at least not in public.

Governments cannot provide for all the needs of the disadvantaged, and large numbers of organizations run by business people work hard to provide extra funds. Unfortunately, many of the same people who spend large sums assisting the disabled carefully avoid close contact with recipients of their largesse. Not all firms are willing to employ people who stutter severely, and the busy captains of industry more often than not respond coldly to handicaps of any kind.

Psychologists, sociologists, and anthropologists have theorized about this paradoxical rejection of handicapped people. Some feel that our society establishes largely material goals, and, in the fight for status, security, and approval, anybody who gets in the way is liable to be trampled underfoot in the impatient mêlée. The corporate urge to help the disabled has been described as an attempt to dissipate the feelings of guilt that arise from maltreating them in the workplace. Rather like running for a bus, pushing a man on crutches into the traffic, and paying someone else to take him to the hospital. Others feel that people who assist the handicapped do so from a feeling of, 'It could happen to me.' It may be that people are simply reluctant to look the harsher realities of life in the face. They push aside the visible evidence, yet want to help at the same time.

Rejections of stutterers by society can be remarkably subtle. Every person who is severely disfluent has experienced the unspoken brush-off by someone who greets him in a friendly, open manner and then, when he blocks, adopts a withdrawn, guarded expression. It may only be a slight change in expression, but it signals that the glass wall is being firmly bolted in place between the stutterer and his audience. When a stutterer becomes more fluent it is quite a shock when this shift in expression doesn't occur.

Surviving childhood and adolescence

The young teacher at the boarding school had little experience of dealing with children who stuttered. His patience was wearing thin as the twelve-year old boy tried to read his part as Brutus in Shakespeare's *Julius Caesar*. Blocking badly on every line, the boy held up the play, and the other children in the class became restless. The teacher suddenly exploded, 'Sit down, you stupid boy! If you haven't the brains to speak you shouldn't be here.'

This happened in several successive classes and the teacher made a point of ridiculing the boy and calling him 'stammer-mouth.' The other students naturally followed his cue. Understandably, the boy became sullen and withdrawn. The teacher eventually went too far, whereupon the youngster stood up, said loudly, firmly, and fluently, 'Unless you stop this and apologize I refuse to answer any more of your questions,' and sat down, dry-eyed but shaking with fury.

He kept his word. Although he spoke to other teachers and students, he ignored his tormentor. When asked a question he looked straight ahead and remained silent. He was taken to the principal, chastised, and repeatedly kept in after school, but he stuck it out until the principal finally told him that the teacher would never apologize. During the lunch break the boy walked out of the school, trudged the twenty miles home, and flatly refused to return. He'd tried the fight response and it had failed, so he took the other alternative, flight.

Was this the action of a disturbed child? Perhaps a better interpretation is that a very angry and determined boy took the only sensible course of action open to him. Incidentally, he did very well at his next school.

Many children who encounter such teachers – and in spite of our enlightenment such individuals still exist – may not have anywhere to escape to, or the will to do so, and their lives can be a misery at school. It is not likely that they will do well scholastically, and their stuttering will probably get worse.

Fortunately, there are some fine teachers with the perception and humanity to look beyond the stutter. I was remarkably lucky. From the age of fifteen to seventeen I came under the wing of David Hodgkinson, a young teacher with whom I shared a fondness for mountains and wild places. He subtly widened my perception and introduced me to literature, poetry, Greek philosophers, the lives of great men, and the intricacies of Bach. Besides providing me with a rich basis upon which to build my life, he managed to persuade other teachers to make allowances for my speech handicap. I was not asked to do the impossible. Unfortunately David died very young, which was a great loss to the young people he could have taught.

Most teachers fall between these two extremes as they struggle to cope with all the different youngsters in their care. Children are expected to conform to certain standards. With increasing dependence on the spoken rather than the written word, students with communication disorders fare badly. For some it is impossible to speak at length during oral examinations, or to give seminars, or to involve themselves in public speaking without the support of effective therapy. If teachers appreciated a stutterer's limitations and permitted him to communicate in other ways, it would relieve the stress. There must be thousands of stutterers who have seen on their school reports, 'Fails to participate actively in the class.' 'Participate' usually means standing up and asking questions, and most people who stutter severely find this very difficult indeed.

If the boy with a stutter is handy with his fists he won't have too much trouble from kids of his own age, although there are always a few bigger boys who will beat him up and continue to taunt. A better approach is to develop an exceptional skill in either the classroom or a sport, particularly the latter, which commands the respect of others. Although I've never enjoyed hunting animals for pleasure, I was a competition-grade marksman from the age of thirteen years. The medals, badges, cups, and other trophies I won reflected well on my peer group and stood me in good stead, relieving some of the pressures and reducing my need to respond aggressively to other kids' jeers about my speech.

People who stutter learn early in life that in order to survive in the classroom, in university, or in a job they must not only be as good as others, but considerably better. Their disability means that they are frequently labelled 'stupid,' and their basic differentness tends to push them outside the herd. They must prove themselves much more than other children.

I learned this at about nine years of age when we were given a written history examination of ten questions. It dealt with the Battle of Hastings in 1066. Nine out of ten of my answers were completely correct, but I blocked badly when we were asked to read our answers aloud and failed the test. Even today I remember my anger and explosive protest to the teacher, who just shrugged her shoulders. As a result I became an 'over-achiever,' and wrote in a letter to my brother, 'I'll show the old cow!'

Most of the severe stutterers I have met who managed to lead full lives had similar experiences. The 'I'll show 'em' belligerence can be exceedingly effective, but it is a two-edged blade that can wound the wielder. Cold-blooded determination to 'show 'em' means that a child does well for the wrong reasons and may derive little pleasure from school achievements beyond a wry, one-in-the-eye satisfaction. I soon realized that my gritted-teeth approach to learning at school was unproductive and relaxed to the point of idleness by thirteen when I realized that I could get good marks by more careful planning and less hard work.

Other severe stutterers in my schools seemed to reach a crossroads at the age of about ten. At that point the impediment either crushed them into inarticulate, lonely unhappiness or began to spin a tough web of determination and single-mindedness throughout their mental fabric. The determined children with stutters became the survivors, but paid the price of excessive stress. Teachers and parents naturally praise the successes of the over-achieving children with partial disabilities, but tend to ignore the tremendous pressure it puts on a child. Perhaps teachers can find ways to reduce the pressures by creating an environment where there is no need for the partially disabled child to 'show 'em.'

The route a child with a stutter follows, whether it be withdrawal or determined achievement, can greatly affect the number of optional courses he takes at school. The children in the regular class get used to a stutterer and cease to bait him after a while, accepting him as a member of their herd. They may even actively support him by helping to fight his battles. Taking optional courses means moving to other groups and meeting new students and teachers. The first few days in a new group can be hell for a stuttering child. It takes sheer guts to expose yourself to it and persist. Children crushed by their stuttering may flatly refuse to take other courses, while the determined stutterer grits his teeth and looks upon the courses and the new situations as challenges – battles to be won. The other people in the new class may find the stutterer edgy and abrasive at first, but this usually disappears as he proves himself, and they accept him. The problem is that a determined child who stutters has to prove himself repeatedly.

It is difficult for a concerned teacher or parent to know what a stuttering child can do and what he cannot do. They may try to avoid exposing the child to situations he cannot handle, but sometimes, with the best of intentions, they underestimate his ability to cope and close doors to his progress. There was a bright senior boy in a school who exhibited leadership qualities, but he was barred from becoming a prefect because the principal felt he would find it hard to maintain discipline. Later in life, still with a stutter, he became a leader and had no difficulty maintaining order. This problem arises in the job situation where the abilities of stutterers to communicate and perform are frequently underestimated by potential employers.

At a time when big is still beautiful in the eyes of some educators, many school classes are still too large for teachers to provide individual attention. If the large classes were broken down into units small enough to allow teachers to educate children and allow for their diversity, partially handicapped children could be given more teacher time. Some schools and teachers insist on oral rather than written communication for certain tests. More flexibility to permit disfluent pupils to communicate in writing would ease pressures. Siphoning off stutterers and other partially handicapped pupils into special classes or schools is not the answer, because young people with partial communicative disorders must learn to perform in the context of society. Isolating them denies them needed opportunities for integration and acceptance.

I never enjoyed the word games and amateur theatricals that other children seemed to find such fun, although at six I played a goblin in a Hallowe'en play and managed to say 'Tonight's the night, aha!' without stuttering. Even today I carefully avoid social occasions where quiz games are played, and I still dislike playing card games involving bidding. All of these involve speaking, and in some games you must speak more quickly than other people to win. I can cope these days, but the games are associated with too many unpleasant memories to evoke pleasure.

Word games, oral spelling, and reciting at junior school were daily nightmares because no allowances were made for my stuttering. This helped to consolidate a minor disfluency into a major, self-reinforcing stutter – although it could have been avoided by a little common sense on the part of the teachers. These days the classroom environment is more enlightened, but a child who stutters is bound to have difficulties where oral performance is rewarded.

Not many people who stutter severely are likely to do well in languages. How I passed my French oral examination is a mystery. My inflexible Latin teacher gave me zero for my reading of Julius Caesar's *Conquest of Gaul*. Gaul was apparently divided into three parts *('Gallia est omnis divisa in partes tres.')*. I managed the *'Gallia est omnis...'* but ground to a halt on *'divisa,'* which, since it was in the first sentence, somewhat truncated the examination.

The child who stutters severely is an oddball in the classroom, and the way others react to this disability may push him even further outside school society. Children enjoy both mental and physical challenges, but a child who stutters may find the impediment such a challenge in itself that he gets fewer kicks out of other activities. I played such games as rugby, cricket, and field hockey well enough, but did not enjoy them or find them a challenge. If you were to climb Everest frequently, the everyday, commonplace hills would be a bore.

Some stuttering children find that they enjoy activities of little interest to the majority (I loved bugs and fossils) and this may alienate their peers. In later life, these unusual interests can be a strength or a weakness depending upon the circumstances. Deep down, most children want to be one of the herd, and this can be very hard for a child with a severe stutter.

Many embarrassing situations can be avoided if teachers give a little thought to planning games that involve speaking. If there is a child who stutters badly in a group, there are often ways of letting him participate without speaking. Teachers should put themselves in the kid's position and try to imagine what it would feel like to have a fifty-fifty chance of blocking on a key word and inviting ridicule. It is tricky, because the child doesn't want to be pushed out of the game, or exposed to disaster. Sometimes it helps just to ask the child what he wants to do.

A stuttering child frequently collects a circle of friends who look beyond the disability and appreciate the person within. I had many intensely loyal friends who took my side against bullies and unpleasant teachers. These good companions were the salt of the earth. Sadly, few of them survived World War II.

When a teacher meets a child it is almost impossible for her to assess what is going on behind the surface mask. I recently looked at pictures of myself as a nine-year-old. The face of the calm-eyed kid with a faint smile completely hid an inner turmoil of anxieties and a burning determination to succeed and survive.

If teachers with stuttering children in their classes would avoid pretending that there isn't a problem and seek qualified advice, it is likely that fewer small children with minor stutters would later develop severe stutters. Even adolescents would have a greater chance of recovering spontaneously or responding to therapy. The classroom may be a jungle, but there is no need for a teacher to be one of the predators.

Living with a stutterer in the family

The attitudes of family members can have as much influence on a stutter as the pressures at school. It seems obvious that a stutterer would feel more relaxed about his speech at home where he knows the people and moves in familiar surroundings, but this is not always the case. During therapy, many stutterers said they found transferring the new speech techniques to the home situation more difficult than using the techniques with strangers in stores. I have always found it exceedingly difficult to use voluntary controlled repetition, prolongation, and cancellation when talking with my three daughters.

The reasons for this anomaly are varied and complex. In my case I feel it is a question of role. We all have images of ourselves acting within a group. Using the speaking techniques creates an unfamiliar person that is just not me – at least, within the family. It needs a great effort to change my identity.

It is easy to be critical of parents who cannot cope with a stuttering child, but most of them do their best. Many stutterers I have known who had severe problems with their mothers and fathers came from well-to-do, upward-striving, middle-class families with materialistic goals. The parents had neither the time nor the patience to worry about their struggling offspring. Other stuttering friends who had bad times came from families where the father was more concerned about his macho image than about his child. The majority of stutterers with parental problems, however, have mothers and fathers who are just nonplussed by the handicap and have no idea what to do about it. If they seek help at all it is generally from the family doctor, who is not always in a position to give good advice about stuttering, however competent he may be in other areas. Some parents just ignore the problem and hope the child will 'grow out of it.' Sometimes the child does, but if I had a stuttering child I wouldn't bet on it.

Sibling rivalry within the family is unavoidable and, as in any other competitive situation, does not involve much compassion. Any weakness is likely to be used in the battles between brothers and sisters. My brother had a large head, size seven and three quarters, and when I was angry I frequently called him 'Big Head.' He replied in kind about my stutter. The no-holds-barred sibling battles were good training grounds for the competitive realities of adult life where the opposition uses any weakness against you.[1]

I was lucky with my family. My brother and sister were not unusually nasty, and I gave as good as I got. A supportive and well-intentioned mother did her best and exposed me to a variety of bad speech therapies – the best available – that helped to turn a mild stutter into a severe one. My father ignored the fact that I stuttered, but did not ignore me. He was a theatre buff, and we went to innumerable shows that entranced a young boy with spectacular performances of the *Student Prince, Chu Chin Chow, White Horse Inn*, and endless Gilbert and Sullivan operettas (compared to which I find modern musicals insipid). I loved to meet the actors in their fancy dress after the shows.

He did the wisest thing he could by exposing me to all types of people and situations. His business friends were a bit dull, but he had financial interests in theatres, circuses, and horses, so I met acrobats and knife-throwers, rode on elephants, played with painted clowns in baggy pants, and rode ponies bareback. It was a small boy's magic world that still brings me happy memories. He took me to the tropics, where he taught me to fish for sharks. He managed to instil in me a self-confidence that stood me in good stead later in life. He was no softie. As an Edwardian father he firmly believed in judicious retribution for all major sins, but he was a better therapist than most of the professionals I met at the time.

People with severe stutters encounter new problems when they acquire families of their own. Most married people I know who stutter severely have been fortunate in their marriage partners. This is not surprising, because any person taking on someone who can hardly speak as a marriage partner must have considerable courage, as well as the more than usual insight it takes to see beyond the tense, disfluent facade and love the person within. Stuttering tends to run in families for reasons that are not fully understood. The non-stuttering partner's parents may not take kindly to having a person with a stutter grafted onto their family tree.

A non-stuttering partner has not only to learn to share the pain that is the stutterer's daily lot, but also to accept the fact that stuttering may limit a person's ability to earn money and provide for the family. A non-stuttering partner had better be a survivor.

Some people who marry disfluent partners don't know what they are letting themselves in for. If they don't have the ability to adapt to the situation, the marriage is liable to disintegrate. I am lucky. My wife, Joan, shares all my problems and looks upon them as a challenge. Before we married, I carefully but nervously laid all the cards on the table and described to her the stresses of living with disfluency. Incredibly, she took me on. Fortunately her parents had met stutterers before, so there was no problem in that area.

The prospect of having children made me distinctly anxious. As an adult I had never hit it off all that well with kids, because their responses to my stutter were unpredictable and sometimes hard to handle. Small children of eight years or less looked wide-eyed and asked honest questions like 'Why do you talk funny?' I handled these by telling them that some people walked in funny ways, or looked funny, and I just talked funny. They usually accepted the explanation. Adolescents were, and still are, more difficult. Some can be very rude and abusive about disfluency and, although it is tempting, it isn't practicable to swat them like irritating blow-flies. I usually resort to my steely-eye-and-chilly-silence routine.

I was aware of the danger that stuttering might develop in our children so, not having access to reliable counsellors, I developed my own approach. There was no hiding the fact that I stuttered severely, but I was careful to show no hint of anxiety or stress about my disfluency. If I blocked I'd say, 'Oops! Better try again!' or laugh when my tongue tangled in a knot. I didn't want the children to associate speaking with stress and fear.

People who stutter severely sometimes feel isolated in the family because they can't read to their children, recite nursery rhymes, or invent stories, but I was determined to communicate using my limited verbal faculties. When the children were very young, my wife and I would read to them in unison, and, occasionally, I fluently told them 'secret' stories in a whisper, which most stutterers can handle. I was always able to sing to them, and car trips were continuous, noisy sing-songs. When my speech was in a good phase I managed to tell them short stories, particularly Kipling's *Just So Stories* ('How the Elephant Got His Trunk' was a great favourite), but I was walking on verbal eggs. As the children grew older and were learning to read, we read slowly together, which was not difficult. When they reached adolescence they preferred television to father's boring stories, so I was able to go off reading duty.

The approach must have worked, because my daughters, who are now adults, have few recollections that I had a speech problem. Even when they reached the age of twenty or more they found it hard to accept that I had difficulties. None of them developed stutters. All of them speak so rapidly and at such great length that I can barely squeeze in a word when we get together.

The wife of someone with severe, uncontrollable stuttering finds herself taking on tasks her husband cannot handle. It makes no sense to be dogmatic about his-and-her roles. If a job involves speaking at length, the guy will need help. The wife of a severe stutterer is likely to find herself doing most of the telephoning. Even today, when I can use the telephone fairly freely, I dislike it to such an extent because of past memories that I tend to leave it to my wife. She's a telephone addict – one of those people who dread the day Bell Canada begins charging for local calls – so she doesn't find it much of a hardship.

When we are outside the house and approach a speaking situation, we decide who will do the talking before we start. From past experience she talks to policemen and customs officers, since they tend to be suspicious of and unpleasant to people who stutter. Some business people are impatient with stutterers, and occasionally my wife deals with them to spare them the fleas they are likely to get in their ears if they were to be obnoxious. Sometimes she deals with government officials, who also tend to respond badly. Dealing with disfluency is not in the regulations.

Sometimes it is hard for a wife to know to what extent she should help. There is always the danger that she will be overprotective, but frank discussion can overcome this kind of difficulty.

Performers, like musicians, who have stutters and become public figures sometimes let their wives read their speeches at social gatherings. The stuttering husband may seem to lean on his fluent wife, but the wife may become dependent on her role as speaker and find it difficult to adapt to the new situation when the stuttering spouse responds to therapy and is able to handle his own affairs. There are many stories of women leaving their husbands when the men became fluent. The wives didn't feel their husbands needed them any more. Maybe the speech challenge was all they had in common.

Living with a stutterer in the family needs understanding and goodwill on both sides. Even without the fractured speech it is not always easy to maintain family harmony.

Friends and lovers

Considering how society treats people with speech disorders, it is amazing that most of the stutterers I meet are warm and friendly people. They may be cautious with strangers and can be a little edgy, but on the whole they are not as withdrawn as most people think.

Some young men with stutters take offence when none is meant. Quite a few people who try to be friendly but nervously giggle when confronted by a stuttering, grimacing youth are fed an undeserved knuckle sandwich. At the age of twenty-three, when my speech was almost completely useless, I was a little explosive myself, and apologized to more than one innocent person after taking great exception to what I thought was ridicule. Fortunately, most people who stutter grow up and become less sensitive. When I am not sure that I'm being ridiculed or patronized, I give the other person the benefit of the doubt. When I am certain that someone is being offensive, my better control of speech and temper enable me to use both carefully chosen syntax and body language, which are much more effective than tapping their claret.

People with stutters can accumulate a circle of valued friends if all concerned are prepared to make the social effort. These friends are exposed to a lesser degree to the same embarrassments, frustrations, and rejections as the stutterer when they are in his company. Only exceptional people can stay the course. At one time when I was in the Armed Forces my speech used to attract trouble like a magnet, and my good, muscular friends helped to save my skin many times.

When a stutterer first meets a stranger the question usually at the back of his mind is: 'How will this person react to my speech?' He may not admit it, but the question is there. Many times I have carried on a friendly, fluent conversation with someone and got along famously until I blocked. Even one block can do it. The person just doesn't want to know you and flees for cover. This used to bother me as a young man, but not any more. Some friends you win and some you lose.

The other side of the picture is that, after the first startled response, some people pull themselves together and persist with the conversation. Sometimes the persistence is sheer curiosity to find out what makes this oddball tick – which is fair enough. When they feel at ease, the merely curious start to ask the kind of questions described in the second chapter of this book. These questions can be genuine or offensive, and the stutterer treats them accordingly. I usually answer unsolicited questions about my speech with stock answers and platitudes until I am sure that the inquiry is genuine. At this point you can usually guess whether or not there will be a future rapport. A stutterer isn't likely to make a friend of a tactless noodlebrain who asks, 'Doesn't it embarrass you when you stutter and people think you are stupid?' My answer to this type of question is, 'Why do you ask that question?' Nevertheless, I welcome genuine inquiries and interest in speech problems.

During these preliminaries, a stutterer feels his way cautiously until both parties are comfortable and can relax, thereby providing a basis for potential friendship. A dialogue is not always sufficient, and acquaintances sometimes fall by the wayside when they share the problems generated by society. The friends who survive these traumatic experiences are pure gold.

The trickiest 'friends' for any handicapped person to recognize and deal with are the patronizers. There are a few people around who, because of their own hidden weaknesses, make friends with the disabled in order to feel better about themselves. Such a relationship can be damaging to a person with a severe stutter, whose self-confidence and self-esteem may not be all that strong, because the patronizer inflates his own ego by subtly putting down the handicapped person. This type of individual can be difficult to recognize. You can't go around questioning everybody's motives. If the 'friend' is upset when the handicapped person can do something better than he can, or makes light of his disfluent companion's successes, there is reason for suspicion. Some lonely stutterers, and other handicapped people whom society has treated cruelly, seek friendship at any price, and they all too easily get into bad company.

It is not advisable to generalize about the relationship between stutterers and members of the opposite sex. Some perfectly normal men with all their faculties in working order find it difficult to establish relationships with women, and vice versa. Stuttering is just another complication in an already complex picture.

It comes as a surprise to many male stutterers when girls reject them for reasons other than their speech. Soon after World War II, I was a member of a university class consisting largely of men who had been battered by war, demobilized early, and sent to college to keep them out of mischief. This influx of mature servicemen increased the competition for university girls to fever pitch, so I focused my attention on the town population.

I developed a passion for a girl who looked like Ava Gardner and worked behind the counter in a pharmacy. My speech was in a bad way, so I was a bit nervous about asking her for a date. I visited the pharmacy several times a week for a month or more and accumulated a vast supply of Ever-Ready razor blades, which were not all that easy to come by at that time. They were all I could afford, and I must have cornered the market. When I summoned enough courage to ask her out she accepted, suggesting that we first have dinner and then go to the local dance hall.

It was our first and last date. She turned out to be a ballroom dancer who had won all kinds of competitions. She said that I danced as though I had three feet. She didn't mind my stuttering in the least, but took the greatest exception to my slow fox-trot. Philosophically, I turned my attention to a girl who also looked like Ava Gardner and worked in a bookstore. She was a Shakespeare buff, and, in spite of my stutter, I managed, by judicious use of the bard's sonnets, to establish a relationship that was entirely satisfactory – until she turned to Chaucer, who was beyond my linguistic ability.

About this time I encountered an attitude that was entirely unexpected. I had a colleague, a cheerful, fair-haired, beefy lad who had been a flying-boat navigator until he was injured. He was not noted for his tact. My stuttering was causing me problems and one day, after I forcibly expressed my feelings about my fractured syntax, he said, 'Don't worry! One day you'll find a girl who can put up with your stuttering and go out with you. Who knows, you might even get married. Anything is possible!' It hadn't entered my head that my disfluency would impede my progress with girls, but he clearly thought that anyone with such a bizarre disability was at the end of the line as far as girl-friends and wives were concerned.

There is no doubt at all that stuttering scares off some young girls, particularly when they are at the age when appearances, normality, and belonging to the in-group are of paramount importance. When young people date they want to feel proud of the companions they introduce to their families and friends. Sometimes a girl with a stuttering boy-friend is forced to make a choice between him and her family, and not many have the strength to withstand that kind of pressure. A pleasant young man in Ontario with a severe, grimacing stutter became firm friends with an attractive girl and accompanied her to many social functions. The girl introduced him to her parents who were perfectly normal farm people. They were polite to the stutterer, but distant. The next time he asked the girl for a date she regretfully turned him down, because her parents had ordered her to get rid of her stuttering friend.

This situation is not uncommon. I went sailing with a girl, but met her father first. He was a practical, down-to-earth business man ('Where there's muck there's money, lad.'), and plainly thought his daughter had brought home a dangerous kook. While we sailed, he had a pair of binoculars trained on us in case I ravished his daughter in the bilges, causing a great deal of on-board hilarity. I solved the problem by looking back with my own binoculars. After a minute or so of staring at each other eyeball to eyeball, he disappeared. I was not asked to stay for dinner.

Some stutterers whose feelings have been trampled and abused by society find it difficult to establish deep relationships with people, particularly those of the opposite sex. They may have many friends and acquaintances, but the relationships move in shallow water, the stutterer being unwilling to go out of his depth and explore the unknown. It is largely a matter of trust. Any deep emotional attachment involves showing another your inner self and assuming the person won't abuse that trust. Some stutterers have inner conflicts that they are not prepared to reveal to others. The disfluent can build their own glass walls for self-protection and never come out into the real world. Sometimes it is up to a friend or lover to break down the walls and establish the trust. You don't have to stutter to have problems about trusting people. Our frenzied society, grasping for monetary will-o'-the-wisps, can be cruel to people with no functional disabilities at all.

The withdrawn stutterer needs to learn to gamble a little, to make mistakes, and to burn his social fingers, accepting that rejection and unkindness are just a part of life. How you deal with them is all that matters. I was saved from withdrawal by an insatiable curiosity about life and people that made me willing to pay the price, however painful, to find out what makes the world tick. Part of me is sociable, and part is solitary. At times I must spend periods alone to recharge my mental batteries. Like other people, stutterers may withdraw for productive purposes, and this has nothing to do with their speech impediments.

People who stutter sometimes avoid social gatherings, and a casual observer may interpret this as shyness or pathological withdrawal. This is not necessarily the case. After talking at work and trying to cope with my stutter, I was usually tired by the end of the day. The last thing I wanted to do was go on talking, however congenial the company. Coping with disfluency can be very tiring indeed, and many stutterers who speak a great deal at the office prefer some non-vocal recreation like swimming, skiing, riding, walking, going to a movie, or engaging in a hobby.

Some stutterers find conversation in large groups difficult, particularly where there is rapid repartee. A disfluent person just cannot get in his word before he is cut off. He finds it impossible to contribute to the conversation, and this can make a chatty social evening very boring. On a few such occasions I have accidentally fallen asleep. Sometimes, to my embarrassment, I have snored loudly.

The academic rat race

There always seemed to be a great many students with stutters when I was at university after World War II – at least one in any group. They all seemed to do well in their examinations. It was easy to conclude that people with stutters are more intelligent than others. While this is incorrect as far as the general population is concerned, there is an element of truth in the case of university students.

University students in the United States and Britain were repeatedly surveyed in the 1930s because most of the speech research was carried out at universities, and the students were convenient to study. Not only were stutterers much more common at American universities (1.8 to 2.8 per cent) compared with the population in general (about 1 per cent), but stuttering university students had consistently higher scores on intelligence tests than fluent students. This apparently superior intelligence possibly reflected the segment of the population at university in those days (upward-striving, middle-class), or the fact that to succeed in school and get into university a stutterer had to be better than others and determined to succeed. Because of difficulties with oral examinations and presentations, the grades of stuttering children tend to be lower than average.[2] The child who gets as far as university must have the wits and the will to beat the odds.

When a person enters university, the highly competitive academic systems make few allowances for a stutter. The student copes or gets out. A severely disfluent student will have a hard time coping with a law course, where oral, Socratic methods of question and answer are used. A disfluent medical student may find it impossible to stand up and describe case histories to a highly critical audience. High grades mean good jobs, and the stutterer had better be a survivor in the more competitive faculties.

I went to universities in Britain at a time when oral seminars and presentations were of minor significance com-

pared with written reports. There are chilling stories of stutterers who went to universities in Europe where all the examinations consisted of standing alone and answering orally
the questions posed by committees of cold-eyed professors.
Stutterers cannot survive in such oral systems. Even today,
most universities in North America require students to give
seminars, whether they stutter or not, even when the subject
is something like forestry, horticulture, or soil science where
verbal disabilities are not likely to be too much of a problem.
I waded my way through a few seminars, oral examinations,
and defences of theses, but it was no joy either to the ex-
aminers or to myself.

The fact that a student who stutters badly cannot cope with
the oral demands of degree courses in subjects like law and
medicine may indicate that the profession is just not for
him. In some cases, however, the methods used in university
faculties prevent a disfluent student from pursuing a career
he could easily manage. Articulacy does not necessarily indicate academic ability.

I was permitted to write when possible, and when I had to
speak I used a variety of visual aids – graphs, charts, and
tables – to minimize the amount of speaking. My colleagues
said they found my talks brief (of necessity), to the point (I
cut out the garbage), and preferable to many presentations by
more wordy peers. This latitude is not available at some
present-day universities, and the oral demands place an unnecessary strain on the disfluent student. The rigidity of
academic, bureaucratic, and governmental institutions is one
of the numerous ills of our time and prevents the varied needs
of individuals being met.

Earning a living: the hidden discrimination

Going for a job interview was as enjoyable for me as visiting
my school principal's study after being found guilty of such a
major transgression as walking with my hands in my pockets.
In both instances I knew that the next few minutes were sure
to be painful.

As a young man I applied for a job breeding raspberries at

a horticultural station in England. I bristled with degrees, know-how, intelligence, and energy, and was shaken when I was defeated by a quiet young woman in thick tweeds and brogue leather shoes. The interviewers were civilized and polite in a reserved British way, and you could see they were trying to remember that the King, God bless him, shared my problem. Nevertheless, it was clear that they had reluctantly concluded that anyone who stuttered as badly as I did couldn't possible have all his marbles. When the kindly, elderly man said I would hear from them, and the tweedy girl was taken to lunch, I knew I'd blown it.

I went through interview after interview, but it was clear that nobody wanted a well-qualified ex-serviceman with a stutter, although they seldom said the stuttering was the problem. Even the fact that I had been to the right kind of school, spoke with the right kind of accent, and knew that you passed a port decanter to the left didn't cut any ice with the establishment. I was astonished therefore when, after a perfunctory interview, I was offered a job growing palm trees by a company making soap and margarine. The salary was four times what I expected, with a house, several servants, an automobile, and six month's leave every two years. My knowledge of palm oil was so limited that I thought copra was something you mined, so I was a little suspicious. Delving into a gazetteer revealed that I was destined for some death hole in the swamps of West Africa where they could put up with my stuttering for the year or so of my life expectancy. I resumed the job hunt.

In retrospect, these depressing interviews were the best thing that could have happened to me. In order to eat I wangled a grant to do research for a post-graduate degree and spent six years on my own talking to deer and pine trees in the Highlands of Scotland, a stutterer's idea of paradise.

Later, with another degree to put on my shingle, I had a further spell of interviews and tried unsuccessfully to get work growing trees in Wales, extracting perfume from lavender in the south of France, and studying water in a waterless part of Australia. Gradually, I learned the art of interviewing and landed a disagreeable job at Oxford University for a few years before embarking on a career of ecological research in Britain's beautiful Lake District where my disability was not much of a handicap.

In spite of all the talk about equal opportunity and civil rights, employers faced with choosing between two people with equal qualifications, one of whom stutters and one of whom doesn't, are likely to select the fluent applicant. In a way this is discrimination, but employers should be able to hire the people they want.

The probationary period is a useful instrument. If employers would give stutterers and other handicapped people a chance to show whether they can handle a job, this would help. If they can't do the job, replacing them is sensible rather than discriminatory. Far too many employers write off an applicant at his first block, forgetting that his speech is likely to be at its worst at a job interview, particularly the hot-seat type of screening where you sit on a hard chair in the middle of a horseshoe of impatient interrogators.

After many painful interviews I learned to act a variety of roles. When the board consisted of bureaucrats, I became a bureaucrat and trotted out the jargon they love, peppering my speech with words and phrases like 'objectives,' 'collective bargaining,' 'decentralization,' 'cost effectiveness,' 'mandatory,' 'critical paths,' 'lines of command,' and 'conceptualization.' With scientists I put on the brilliant-but-eccentric act; and with business people I became a thrusting executive, obsessed with cash flow, rates of return, cost effectiveness, and linear programming. My performances were so effective that people forgot the stuttering and began to offer me jobs.

I was playing roles. Therapists may frown at role-playing to achieve better fluency, but I'd have danced the part of the Sugar Plum Fairy to get a good job.

I was lucky. I had the education and the skills, and my family could house and feed me while I hunted for work. Not all stutterers are so fortunate.

There is no doubt that in the job market there is a great deal of hidden discrimination against people with severe stutters, quite apart from their actual fitness for the work. Stutterers make some people feel uncomfortable. They may not fit in a work group, either because of their stuttering or their tendency to over-achieve and compete aggressively. Employers wanting a contented work force tend to get rid of the odd man out, and it is their prerogative, since they pay the bills. Nevertheless, it would help if employers appreciated what a disfluent person can do rather than what he cannot do. People with stutters and other handicaps can do first-class work. They are often great planners and strategists – they have to be to survive – and this can be an asset.

Stuttering makes you resourceful. You instinctively think about things that could go wrong and devise ways of dealing with them before they happen. A simple problem like having the car break down in a remote area and trying to get help can be traumatic. You walk up to a farm and knock on the door. Someone opens it and at your first block is liable to slam it in your face. If you get as far as the telephone you're likely to block, and the person on the other end may hang up on you. The disfluent and stranded traveller has to sit down and think of a solution. I always carried a pad, a pencil, and a small tape recorder.

People can cope with most things if they curb their urge to take flight. I had just driven to Quebec City when I received a message telling me to represent Canada at an international meeting in the southern United States concerning a subject about which I knew very little. There were no briefings, no guidelines, no time to do any homework, and no allowance for my disability. I just had to be there. An hour before the meeting I alternated between feeling sick and numb, but when I entered the room and adopted the role of government scientist, all the tension disappeared. I blocked and stuttered, but my eccentric-scientist act saved the day. The meeting went remarkably well, and the bottle of Jack Daniel's sour mash in my room soon quieted my jangled nerves. At the time it never entered my head that even a fluent person would have been nervous when faced by such a challenge.

There is no easy solution to the problems stutterers encounter in looking for and keeping jobs. It is necessary to be realistic, but a greater attempt to be open about the problem and deal with it honestly instead of pretending it isn't there would benefit all concerned.

Foreign travel

A few years ago an intelligent, slightly built young man with fair hair set out from Canada on a private adventure, hitch-hiking across Europe and Asia Minor to Afghanistan. He managed to reach his destination and to return home all in one piece. This still amazes me, because he had a very severe stutter and distorted his face as he struggled to speak.

My stutter has landed me in trouble many times on my travels. Customs officers are the worst. I suppose they look for signs of anxiety and tension in guilty passengers carrying contraband. When my stutter was in a bad phase I probably gave the impression of being agitated when all I was doing was trying to say 'I've nothing to declare.' Once, on returning to Britain from a visit to a research laboratory in the Netherlands and being asked by the customs officer if I had anything to declare, I blocked on the word 'No.' He passed my bags; however, when I was leaving the building an official in plain clothes hustled me into a nearby office where, in more ways than one, they left no stone unturned as they looked for diamonds. I was interrogated at gun point at the border between France and Italy because I blocked. In New York's Kennedy Airport a cold-eyed lout in uniform opened and up-ended my suitcase, scattering belongings everywhere, looking in the linings, and saying, 'What are you so nervous about?' and ignoring my explanation that I was not nervous, I just stuttered. Spanish customs officers in Madrid were suspicious, snarky, and belligerent about my disfluency, but they were like that with everybody.

Even entering Canada from the United States was a problem. If I blocked when I answered the customs officer's questions, my car was sure to be pulled over and searched. There were exceptions, and some customs officers were helpful and courteous. In one of the banana republics, where customs officials are over-officious, blocking severely could mean mouldering in a rat-infested dungeon for years.

Trying to cope with a foreign language is bad enough without a stutter. When I was in Italy I fluently asked a young woman in a store for Virginia cigarettes to avoid smoking their acrid Nationales. I had looked up the words in my little Italian dictionary and couldn't understand the shouting and fist-shaking that followed my request – until someone told me I'd muddled the grammar and asked the girl if she were a virgin.

A stutterer will experience abroad all the problems he meets at home, but on a bigger scale because of the language barrier. Asking for food in restaurants and merchandise in stores in a foreign language can be traumatic even for fluent people, as many Americans find when they visit Quebec City thinking it's the same as New Orleans. Taxi drivers can be a pain. Some try to charge you double fare if they think you can't or won't argue (I can and do!).

I like seeing new places, meeting new people, and participating in new cultures, but for me travelling has never been as enjoyable as other people seem to find it. For many years I travelled all over the world on business, and now that I don't have to do so it is something of a relief. I was offered an interesting short-term job in Paris a year or so ago, but turned it down because I couldn't bear the thought of battling in French with hotels, taxi drivers, and officials for three months. Some severe stutterers love travelling and don't seem to mind the hassle.

Stores and restaurants

The majority of people take speaking, like their heartbeats, for granted. If they want something, they ask for it. If they want to ask a question, they ask it. If they want to protest, they protest. A stutterer never takes speech for granted even in his fluent phases. He may have had good therapy, but he must always watch his way of speaking and plan for possible failures. Stutterers can ask for things, question, and protest, but, like porcupines making love, only with the greatest care.

Stores and restaurants present a severe stutterer with a multitude of problems. Store clerks vary in their responses, but many are hostile and some are downright rude. In some restaurants if you stutter at the headwaiter when you arrive he is liable to try to fob you off with a table between the washrooms and the kitchen door if you let him – which I don't. As a young man I just pointed at the menu for dishes I wanted to order and even acted mute to avoid unpleasantness from the waitress. Many times I ordered dishes I didn't want because they were easy to say. I still can't ask for pressed duck.

When my speech was very bad indeed I was completely lost without my pencil and scribbling pad, because I couldn't order anything in a store without writing it down. Occasionally, I encountered someone who was blind or couldn't read, which really put gravel on my gears. After countless bad experiences in these situations, I found trying to use speech techniques in stores and restaurants incredibly difficult, but these situations cause me few difficulties today.

Public transport

Public transport is not usually a major problem for severely disfluent people unless they have to ask for directions or tell the driver where to go in front of other passengers. Airport buses can be a trial because the drivers stand up at the front and ask for destinations. If the name of the hotel is difficult to say I am in trouble, particularly if it's in French. Taxis used to be difficult. Even if I wrote the address on a piece of paper, the driver would ignore it and ask where I wanted to go. If I had trouble speaking, the drivers were less than polite, and I was not all that tolerant of their bad manners.

Railway trains were fine. You got your ticket, sat in your seat, and shut up. Nobody bothered you. Air travel can be tricky; it depends on whom you get beside you. Some passengers are a delight to talk to, like the very old lady in her eighties who, when I was in my mid-forties and doing calculations on a pad, leaned over and said, 'You'll be one of them young students!' and told me about her adventures as a nurse in the Arctic fifty years ago.

Passenger aircraft are full of young executives who read too many books on psychology and tend to suffer from verbal incontinence and impertinent curiosity. They ask questions like, 'Is it true that all people with communication disorders have castration complexes?' unaware that my wishful thinking about them includes more than a complex in their futures. I avoid sitting next to young men with expensive brief-cases, manicured finger-nails, Holt Renfrew pin-stripes, glossy shoes, and dollar signs glittering in their eyes.

Hotels

Hotels that are large and expensive frequently have well-trained staffs that are used to dealing with eccentric and even objectionable people. If you spend money and don't muck up the room, set the place on fire, pinch the towels, or offend the other guests, you are welcomed with open arms. They won't mind if you're a stuttering Martian with seven legs provided you have the right credit card. If you stutter and offer to pay with real money, then you're in deep, deep trouble ...

The arrival part is not too bad. Even if I blocked badly on my name at the reception desk I could always shove my credit card under their noses so they could identify me. The difficulties arose when I reached my room and wanted to take advantage of the hotel's services. You ask for most services by telephone. That darned telephone!

I stayed at hotels for twenty years before I used room service. I was so disfluent and conditioned to block on telephone calls that if I wanted a maintenance man to repair a leaky faucet, I just put up with the drip. It was no use going down to the desk and asking for a plumber. They just referred me to room service. So the tap dripped. Ordering meals or drinks in my room was impossible, so I invariably ate elsewhere. Asking for an early call on the phone by giving the room number and the time was out of the question, so I learned to carry an alarm clock. Making a long-distance call through the hotel operator was a major battle. First you had to give your name and room number, and then the digits. I usually ground to a halt on my name until the operator cut me off. The family learned not to expect calls from me when I was away, but some business calls were unavoidable. My speech was usually not bad once I connected with my target, but the process of getting there was exhausting.

I learned to use verbal aids. I could, if I spoke with great care, tape messages on my own, so I bought a small tape-recorder and recorded what I wanted to say to the operator, with two repeats in case she didn't hear the first time. I lifted the receiver, dialled the operator, played the tape to get over the vital message of name, room, and number, and ad libbed from then onwards. It took a bit of practice, and I once played the operator a recording of the Glasgow Orpheus Choir by mistake, making matters worse by going off into peals of laughter. But usually it worked remarkably well.

The staff of many small hotels run as family businesses are most courteous and helpful, and these hotels can be gems. The best we ever stayed at nestled in the middle of a peach orchard in Pennsylvania, near to the village with the unusual name of Intercourse. The Amish people who ran the place were not in the least put out by my stuttering, and we spent a tranquil night in spite of the bangs of the bird-scarers. In contrast, many of the cantankerous receptionists at dingy dumps in the boondocks are incredibly unpleasant to fluent customers and intolerable if you block. After a preliminary effort to be polite, it is sometimes necessary to be outspoken. The angrier I used to get, the more fluent I became. With my vast vocabulary of synonyms that I used to substitute for difficult words, I managed to make my feelings known, stutter or no stutter. If you have trouble speaking, this kind of hotel usually makes you pay in advance and may not accept your credit card. Nevertheless, I prefer to stay at small places rather than those twenty-storey monsters in which you fry to a crisp if some fool smokes in bed and sets the place alight.

I used to get angry with rude receptionists, but now I just feel sorry for them. They are just tired, bored, afraid of the unfamiliar, and behave in the only way they know.

It would help even in the best hotels if a person who has difficulty speaking could go to the information desk and ask for room service or an early call. The major hotels are proud of their facilities for the handicapped, including ramps for wheelchairs, specially designed washrooms, and chains and pulleys to help a person get into and out of bed and the bath. This is fine, but there are handicapped who have no trouble using their limbs. No allowance is made for the stutterers, the aphasics, the deaf, and the mute who, once in their rooms, tend to be trapped by the glass walls of their handicaps. Hotels can be lonely places.

In the near future we are likely to see telephones in homes and hotels linked to computer terminals, video displays, and printers. I envy the stutterers of the future who will be able to key-punch their messages to room service or the information desks without struggling to speak. A room or two in a hotel with a computer link would make the stay much more enjoyable for those with speech and hearing disabilities.

The telephone nightmare

To a greater or lesser extent, the telephone haunts all people who stutter. The mere sight of the instrument can recall a multitude of humiliations. The ring of a telephone that needs answering can arouse sheer panic. I discovered to my surprise that a great many people with normal speech are scared by the telephone, and that most callers become exceedingly nervous when an answering machine asks them to leave a message. Stuttering just amplifies the fears.

The telephone is such an impersonal way of communicating. You can't see the speaker and read the body language that plays such a large role in a stutterer's communication. The telephone message is conveyed by mere words. There may be information in the tone of voice, but the spoken words are the main thing.

When I stuttered very badly I'd pick up the phone, dial the operator, and try to say the number. I inevitably blocked, and more often than not she'd say, 'Please put your telephone down and dial again. We have a bad connection.' cutting me off before I could explain that it was me, not the phone, that had a bad connection. This was repeated three or four times until I bellowed, 'Hold it a minute, god damn it! Keep the plug in and listen!' This I could say fluently if I was mad enough. When I had all her attention, I tried to say the number careful digit by careful digit, but there were long silences between syllables. She never got the number right the first time, so I battled through the digits over and over again. Some valiant souls stayed the course, but many operators hung up in despair. For me the telephone was not a practical form of communication. I coped at the office, but didn't willingly make a social call for twenty-five years.

In Britain most of the operators were polite; at the worst they were impatient. My most memorable call was to a rural exchange near the resort of Os in Norway. The male operator's English was non-existent and my Norwegian was tourist gibberish, but I managed to read the carefully rehearsed digits from my dictionary. Of course I blocked; it still amazes me how any Scandinavians get their tongues around their vowels. The man became abusive, so I put down the telephone and looked up in my dictionary a few of the words he had used. Most of them referred to the nether parts of farmyard animals so I carried out more careful research. I dug from the dictionary a few choice Norwegian nouns and adjectives about unlikely ancestry, picked up the phone, dialled, and fluently returned his serve. Match and game. I never did make the call.

In France, Italy, and Spain telephoning was impossible. I could say the words with a passable accent, but when I hesitated the blast of grapeshot that came over the wire would put anybody off.

North American responses are patchy. In New York State and Massachusetts the operators are so impatient that they don't seem to be able to cope with people who stutter, or anybody else for that matter. Soft-spoken operators in Georgia are wonderful. They just wait patiently until the number emerges and even have a chat afterwards, hoping that I enjoy their fair state.

Canada is a country of contrasts, and this applies to telephone operators. In British Columbia, Alberta, and Saskatchewan, they generally treat my disfluency with the greatest courtesy and patience; even in Ontario a stutterer using the phone will have few problems west of North Bay. The nearer you get to Ottawa, the harder it is for a stutterer to use Ma Bell's facilities. Maybe it's the feisty, Gallic temperament, but as soon as I hear an operator with a French accent I think, 'Here we go again!' I had no problems at all when I stuttered in both English and French while I worked in Quebec, except on the telephone.

One young man stuttered when he contacted an Ottawa

operator. Following the guidelines of his therapy he paused and said to the operator, 'I have a stutter. I shall probably repeat words, and pause. Please hold on!' To his amazement the male operator began to jeer at him and imitate his speech, so the stutterer lost his temper and slammed down the phone. He should have asked for the supervisor and reported the incident, but even if he had done so it's doubtful that it would have done much good. I've reported abusive operators several times. Only once did I get a reply, and the letter just made polite, placatory noises.

It is a mystery to me why some operators respond this way. As a rule a person's reaction to stuttering seems to be rooted in fear, so maybe the operators are scared of not being able to cope with a stutterer; or perhaps they mistake him for a drunk. Bell has expressed concern for the handicapped and has devised electronic equipment to help disabled people to use the telephone more easily. I just wish they'd take a closer look at the human factor and teach more of their operators good manners and how to deal with callers who cannot speak very well. It's not too hard. Just wait. The words will come eventually.

Even telephoning can be funny. I was taking therapy in Ottawa and was at the stage when you deliberately repeat every first sound three times (voluntary controlled repetition). I wanted a long-distance number, and there was no direct dialling, so I contacted the operator and fluently said, 'Six, six, six, one, one, one, three, three, three, five, five, five,' until I heard choking sounds on the line and realized what I was doing. I burst out laughing, explained the problem, and we both enjoyed the joke.

Despite lighter moments and even with improved fluency, I dislike the phone. The rude, impatient responses of some of the operators to even minor pauses and disfluencies still raise my hackles. Until the entire system is automated, and a person with a stutter can dial all numbers, the only answer is better education for the operators.

I often wonder what the snarky ones look like. When they put video screens on the phones I may be surprised to find that some of them don't sit pulling the wings off wriggling, helpless flies.

The faceless bureaucracy

Bureaucrats tend to manage their affairs by the rule books, and there don't seem to be any guidelines about how to deal with the vocally disabled. Managing employees who differ from average is a human problem, and the last concern of all the government regulations I have read seems to be the problems of humanity. Give the public service an administrative riddle to solve and it will succeed – expensively, perhaps, but nevertheless succeed. Give the service a human problem and it will flunk the test.

The Income Tax Office in Ottawa has facilities for the handicapped, but when you enter the advisory room, you take a number. When you are called, you stand in a kind of cattle stall facing a flinty-eyed tax officer behind a plastic counter. You can't sit, but stand like a penitent so that all the waiting victims can hear your financial confessions. Imagine that you have a stutter and block on every fourth word. You try to explain your tax problem in the bureaucratic bafflegab that is the only language the clerks understand. It's hard enough for a fluent person to cross this hurdle, but for a stutterer it can be a nightmare. All the supplicants behind you hear your blocks and repetitions and get an earful about your problems of cash flow. You lose your privacy and dignity as well as your money. Why can't they provide the privacy of cubicles with four walls?

At the Passport Office the person behind the counter tends to get difficult if you block, and the rigmarole of swearing in for citizenship is about as hard for a stutterer as taking marriage vows. In any government office you meet, besides the usual bureaucratic shell-game, blank-eyed unhelpfulness when you block. Some people with stutters find the bureaucracy easier to deal with than others, but most people who stutter very badly tell a sad tale of rudeness and obstruction. Fluent people get the same run-around, but a stutter makes the problem worse.

The move to bilingualism in Canada has placed many civil servants who stutter in a difficult position. They may have done a good job for years, but the regulations demand that public servants in management positions or who deal with the public be proficient in French. Whether you see a franco-phone once every two years is beside the point. Many older people find it hard to learn French – which is why the lists of executives in the federal government telephone books read like the Paris directory – and many stutterers find the oral methods used in language schools impossible to handle. The language regulations virtually bar employees with severe stutters from promotion to more senior positions they could handle efficiently.

By fancy administrative footwork I managed to avoid the French courses and still get promoted, but many disfluent employees are less fortunate and are limited by blind application of discriminatory regulations. More flexibility in the language program to allow for the fact that some employees have linguistic problems would at least indicate a little concern for the people involved. There's not much hope that the situation will change in the near future because, as L.J. Peter wrote, 'a bureaucracy defends the status quo long past the time when the quo lost its status.'[3]

The arm of the law

It was difficult to drive in the rush hour on the ice-covered, granite cobblestones of Aberdeen, Scotland, without sliding into other vehicles, and I cursed the police car when it abruptly cut in front and signalled me to stop. A red face framed by a chequered police cap peered suspiciously in at the window sniffing for evidence of alcohol and asked if I knew that one of my rear lights had blown and that travelling without all my lights was breaking the law. I promised the policeman I would go to a mechanic on the way home. Unfortunately, 'm' is difficult for me to say and I blocked badly on 'mechanic.' I was promptly arrested and carted off to the cop shop where I had the devil of a time convincing the law that I was sober.

Police tend to associate disfluency with drunkenness, and before the breathalyser tests it was hard for a stutterer to prove that he was sober. Earlier in this century, the test for drunkenness was to walk a straight line and reel off tongue-twisters like, 'The Leith police dismisseth us.' A person who stuttered was sure to fail the test. A great many people were detained merely because they tangled their words.

About the time of my arrest a well-known scientist found himself in a British court. He was brilliant, one of those academicians who seemed to be good at everything. His lucid pen described physics, mathematics, and mechanics in a manner everybody could understand and enjoy. Like many exceptional people he was eccentric, and when he spoke he bumbled. He was so inarticulate that he was hard to understand. The police arrested him in his car in London. Although he was stone cold sober, a charge of drunken driving stuck as far as the courts, where it was dismissed when witnesses testified that he always spoke that way.

As a young man I was detained twice for stuttering. In addition, because of my impediment, I have had difficulties with the police so many times that I've lost count. Police deal with the seamy side of life and tend to be suspicious of anybody who acts in a way that is outside their usual experience. I now realize that many police in North America are frightened by unfamiliar situations and unusual people. A lone New York State police trooper stopped to find out why our car, which had conked out, was parked beside the turnpike in the pouring rain. He was plainly terrified when I blocked badly, and he became belligerent, virtually accusing me of stealing my own car.

There are many fine police officers (and I knew one policeman who stuttered and had quite a time in court), but on the whole I avoid contact with the law. The odds are too high that there will be unpleasantness. The police have the guns and the law on their side, and a stutterer is likely to come off second best in any altercation.

The only way to solve this problem is for the police to be taught that about 1 per cent of the population stutters and that there are many others – stroke victims with aphasia, clutterers, people with cleft palates, and the totally deaf – who speak in strange ways that are sometimes hard to understand. Altogether there must be five million people in North America who, for one reason or another, have difficulty speaking, and the majority of these are respectable, lawabiding citizens. There is no need for the police to give them a hard time.

I knew two pretty girls who were totally mute, but who both had boy-friends and managed to lead fairly normal lives. I asked them if they had encountered any problems with the police, and they both replied, in writing, that although they had met officers there had been no trouble at all. On my next encounter with the police, I pretended to be mute and wrote my answers to their questions on a pad. It worked, and the tough-looking officers were courteous and helpful. It seems to be all right if you shut up but far from all right if you talk in a strange way. I was tempted to remain mute in future encounters, but you can't go around acting false roles all the time.

In the days when I stuttered very badly I avoided the courts at all costs and was reluctant to appear as a witness. This attitude arose from my experience of court proceedings in Britain when I was in the Armed Forces. We were granted week-end passes to the nearest town, and during a night out with the boys my money ran out as the beer poured in – our pay was only two pounds a week at the time. Rather than sit in draughty Church Army canteens or read uplifting books sitting on hard chairs in Salvation Army hostels, I used to watch the court proceedings. It was the cheapest show in town.

At two of the sessions stutterers were involved. One stutterer was accused of child abuse, and the prosecution's lawyer used the defendant's inarticulacy as evidence that he had mental problems, was an unreliable member of society, and could have committed the crime. The objections by the defence were disallowed by the judge. The trial went on for several days, so I never heard the outcome, but it was a gross misinterpretation of the implications of stuttering.

At another session, the main witness for the defence, was a quiet, shy, wispy-haired little man who stuttered badly. The prosecution's lawyer fired questions at him rapidly, and the poor guy's speech gradually fell apart. The lawyer implied that the stutterer was not mentally equipped to be a competent witness ('M'lud, the witness seems unwilling or unable to reply to questions pertinent to the case'), and the witness was dismissed.

The figure of justice has a sword in one of her hands, and the legal profession is not noted for its humanity. In most courts the opposing barristers are adversaries, and in this competitive situation no holds are barred provided they are legal and comply with the regulations that govern court proceedings. Any weaknesses of the defendant, plaintiffs, and witnesses are exploited by the battling lawyers. A stutterer can come off very badly indeed.

Judges and barristers should realize that people who stutter are, apart from their speech, average citizens. It should be possible for a person with a communication problem to reply in writing or other ways suited to his handicap. There are indications that courts dealing with the rights of spastics and other impaired citizens permit unusual forms of communication, and this is a step in the right direction.

I never liked the idea of justice being blindfolded, because it implies that justice relies only on what it hears. What you hear from disfluent people can give the wrong impression, and it is necessary to open your eyes and look more deeply to get at the facts. Aristotle once said that the law is reason free from passion. Unfortunately it is also free from compassion in too many cases.

The two masks of the media

When I went to the theatre as a small boy I was fascinated by the plaster reproductions of early Greek theatrical masks that decorated the frieze above the stage. In most theatres there were two masks, one a laughing face representing comedy, and the other a face with the mouth and eyes distorted by grief representing tragedy. I learned later that theatrical comedy can be tragic and that the two masks cannot always be separated.

Writers, artists, and actors who entertain the masses mould public opinion for good or evil. Today television and the cinema wield enormous power. For thousands of years authors and actors have cashed in on the idea that audiences find disabilities funny, further reinforcing this point of view by their performances.

When the Roman Empire was at the peak of its power, a man called Balbus Blaesius was locked in a cage beside the Appian Way, the main thoroughfare to Rome. He had a very

severe stutter and was only one of many disabled unfortunates on exhibition for the entertainment of passers-by. For
a small coin Balbus would talk to wayfarers and delight them
with his tangled tongue. Inhuman? Certainly, but the exhibition was part of a long tradition of poking fun at handicapped and misshapen people.

We are supposed to be more enlightened today, but a few
years ago I watched a television show about a fair where one
of the main attractions was a young man with cluttering, stuttering speech who earned his living by shrilly mangling his
words for the paying public in the tradition of Balbus
Blaesius in his cage. At these fairs people still pay to see
dwarfs and bearded ladies, just as I used to pay my sixpence
to see two-headed snakes and five-legged calves when I was a
small boy fascinated by the incongruities of the world.

It is difficult to understand how adults can derive entertainment from looking at or listening to people with disabilities. It is too easy to say that people are basically sadistic.
It is more likely that they think, 'Thank goodness it's not
me.' Maybe that is why people go to see the deformed and
disfluent – relieved thankfulness.

Open ridicule of handicapped people in movies and on
television is not common today, but there are frequent implications that people who stutter are foolish, mentally
retarded, or psychopathic. In many movies, a weak but
sinister character is given a stutter to illustrate his psychopathic tendencies, and an actor playing a sadistic killer may
well stutter to imply an unhappy childhood that caused his
mental disturbance. Most of the characters on the media who
stutter are portrayed as weak, stupid, and unreliable – as
cowards, wimps, or dangerous criminals – and people begin
to get the idea that this is the way things are.

Comedians can't help cracking jokes about a person who
stutters, or who is deaf, or who has a wooden leg, but there
are ways of doing it. Stutterers, deaf people, and those with
wooden legs can get into some funny situations. Few of these
people would object if people laugh *with* them. But none
likes being laughed *at*. Jokes about people who are different
can be fairly harmless. It depends upon the context. Canadians joke about 'Newfies,' Americans about 'Polacks,' the

English about the 'Micks,' and the Australians about 'Poms,' and the inferences are that the butts of the jokes are simple or stupid. I don't much like these jokes, but mostly they lose their sting because people know that the targets are anything but stupid. With a stutterer or deaf person they are not so sure, because the difficulty in communicating may suggest stupidity.

Jokes that imply that handicapped people are stupid are in poor taste, and also somewhat cowardly, since the target is seldom in a position to retaliate. Nevertheless, people should retaliate more. Whenever I see, hear, or read in the media suggestions that disfluent people are stupid, unreliable, or psychopathic I write letters pointing out the errors and the implications. I must have written hundreds of such letters, but have never had a reply. If more people expressed their distaste, the media might eventually get the message.

Disabilities are not funny. There are so many other ways of entertaining people that it shouldn't be too hard to cease the implied ridicule. In recent years, a few TV shows have handled stuttering unusually well. I remember one about a young boy with a stutter who fell in love with his school counsellor. The difficult topic was handled sensitively, with gentle humour. In another program a talk-show producer with a stutter addressed his staff using excellent word prolongation, cancellation, and easy onset. The script writer and producer knew their jobs.

More often, however, the implication is that anybody who stutters is an idiot. Many comedians seem to go along with Will Rogers's averral that everything is funny as long as it happens to somebody else, but Aesop put it better when he wrote, 'Clumsy jesting is no joke.'

Acceptance: the two-way transaction

There is no doubt that some stutterers deliberately withdraw from society, either because of the great effort it requires to speak or because of society's treatment of them. Unfortunately, as Shakespeare wrote in *Cymbeline*, 'Society is no comfort to one not sociable.' Unless the stutterer is willing to make the effort, however painful, he cannot expect people to accept him and co-operate with him. Neither can people expect the disfluent to become useful citizens unless individuals make the effort to calm the irrational fears that arise when confronted by a grimacing person trying to force his way through a speech block. These fears are the foundation of the glass wall that separates stutterers from other people. Acceptance is a two-way transaction. Society won't accept handicapped people unless these people are willing to be accepted.

Some people who stutter have been so battered by society that asking them to come out of their den to meet their tormentors and establish productive links is, in the stutterer's eyes, like asking a deer to hold a meeting with a pack of wolves. It may take time for the stutterer to develop trust and be assured of the new and unfamiliar goodwill. Some people with severe stutters live in a fairly hostile world because their mode of speech makes people nervous. Others find the world more benign; it depends upon the circumstances and the social circles in which they move.

There are no set rules about how to break down the walls between the disabled and society, but good starting points are patience, good manners, goodwill, and a desire to look beyond superficial appearances. Unfortunately, patience is rare in a busy world, many people look upon good manners as redundant, and the media have persuaded people to value superficial appearances rather than intrinsic qualities.

The stutterer himself must accept that employers have their likes and dislikes and are, to some extent, free to indulge them. Not all those who reject members of minority groups are bigots. An employer may have hired several people from the Outer Hebrides before, and if they gave him a bad time he's not likely to be enthusiastic about employing another of them. He forms his opinion and preferences on experience – incomplete perhaps, but experience none the less – and this is not necessarily prejudice. A person with a stutter, a paraplegic, a black person, or a woman, any of whom may have been rejected by an employer, should be sure of the facts before crying, 'Prejudice!'

Government institutions, in particular, need to take off their bureaucratic blinders, look beyond the regulations, and accept that blindness, deafness, and limb malfunction are not the only disabilities. In Canada, the income-tax department insists that people are only disabled for the purpose of income-tax deductions if they are blind or spend most of the day in a wheelchair or in bed. People who manage to get around painfully on prosthetic devices or crutches are not usually permitted to deduct the expenses they incur in over-coming their disability so that they can earn a living. An academic whose hands were so crippled with cerebral palsy that he could not write was not allowed to deduct from his taxable income the cost of hiring a secretary to type for him. People dragging their legs around on crutches were not per-mitted to use the handicapped tax deductions. The irony is that this bureaucratic brutality takes place within a federal organization that also contains a Department of Health and Welfare dedicated to helping the sick and disabled.

Trying to change the legislative and bureaucratic status quo is reminiscent of the Greek legend about poor old Sisyphus, who was forever condemned to roll a huge stone up a hill, with the stone always rolling back just before he reached the top. Getting past the bureaucratic fortifications can be frustrating. You get to the right person in one branch and he passes the buck to another branch. The Sisyphean toil is repeated on many hills and you seldom get anywhere unless you find a politician with the key that fits all the bureaucratic doors, or better, a hammer to bash them down.

Stutter power

A tall young man walked along the beach of an Ontario resort wearing a dark blue T-shirt with 'Stutter Power' writ-ten in yellow across the front. Clearly he had no hang-ups about revealing his disability to the whole world, but unfor-tunately the words were wishful thinking. Stutterers have little power to change the attitude of society or to end discrimination in the job market.

The harsh fact is that most stutterers find it hard to stand up in public and protest. If they tried they wouldn't be taken seriously because society has been conditioned to ridicule stuttering. If circus clowns were being discriminated against and appeared on television to state their case with painted, sad faces and bulbous noses, they wouldn't get much support. People would just laugh.

There are many organizations that help the physically and mentally disabled, the blind, the deaf, and the mute to get jobs and deal with discrimination. Unfortunately, nobody seems to help the *partially* disabled. Crippled people who get around without a wheelchair and try to earn a living, kids with very limited vision who press their thick glasses close to their school books, those with hearing that is so poor that hearing-aids only help a little, and the people with speech distorted by cleft palates, stutters, and stroke-induced aphasia get little consideration or help.

A young man at a reputable Canadian high school had a severe problem with his vision. He was not totally blind, but he was a slow reader and lived in a misty world that was always out of focus. At school he was poor at games and did not get high grades, so he was continually teased and punched by other kids and scolded by teachers for his slowness. His life at school was a misery. A few years ago his parents convened a meeting with an eye specialist, the school principal, and the boy's teachers. Few of the teachers bothered to turn up, and shortly afterwards the boy dropped out of the school system. Only his parents were willing to stand up and give him support. He wasn't totally blind, so nobody cared.

Even when partially disabled people go to see an ombudsman or other authority concerned with civil rights they are not likely to get much help, because the official may well hold the general view that partial disabilities do not cause people much distress. The idea of a militant stutterer may seem ludicrous to many, but it is high time the disfluent learned to speak out or get someone to speak for them.

Stutterers have formed self-help groups, particularly those which help people with stutters to maintain their better speech. Most of these groups are offshoots from the speech clinics. There have been attempts to form lay stuttering associations in Canada to express stutterers' viewpoints and promote their rights, but most fade away from lack of support. There are several successful, active groups in the United States, but few of the groups are militant.

Stutterers are a silent minority, generally avoiding public

exposure and finding it difficult to work on committees or function in large groups. Perhaps the huge numbers of people who stuttered at some time in their lives but later became fluent could co-operate with the disfluent to present their case more forcibly. They could put over the idea that there are more handicaps than being in a wheelchair or being deaf or blind, and that stuttering and other partial disabilities can cause people real hardship.

If there were legal and financial support, class actions could be brought against media people who condone or foster the idea that people who stutter are psychopathic or mentally incompetent. These slanders and libels reduce stutterers' opportunities in the job market. An organization that is not fearful of retaliation from the income-tax department could present a strong case for permitting stutterers and others with partial disabilities to deduct the costs incurred in hiring the help and purchasing the apparatus (tape recorders, maskers, assistants, transport, etc.) that help them earn a living.

During the seventeenth century Pascal wrote, 'The property of power is to protect.' If people with stutters feel they need more protection, they should persuade more articulate people to support them and use the power of group representations.

The elderly stutterer

There was an old farmer who enjoyed sitting on the front porch smoking his pipe and looking out at his fields and barns where he used to work so hard. He had stuttered badly all his life. A friend he hadn't seen for many years called in for a chat, and they walked over the farm talking about old times. The friend was astonished at the man's fluency. 'What happened to your stutter?' he exclaimed. 'Oh that,' the farmer smiled. 'These days I'm too old and tired to bother with stuttering. It's no trouble at all.'

There are several versions of this story, and they may all be apocryphal, but the tale illustrates an important point. Stuttering, the fighting to speak, is hard work. It takes youth and energy to wrestle the words into submission. Fighting to speak is so tiring that you only willingly talk at length when you are trying to make your way in the world, meet challenges, fight for acceptance, and scale life's pinnacles in spite of the verbal odds stacked against you. All this struggling inflates the tensions and anxieties that make the stutter worse in the distressing spiral of untreated disfluency.

In old age there is no longer the drive to succeed at your job and climb the corporate ladders. It's hard enough dealing with life's level ground without tackling the challenges of the heights. You let go a little and look back, maybe with a chuckle or two, at the enormous amount of effort you spent tilting at the windmills of your imagination, fighting adversaries that were really yourself, and seeking Holy Grails that turned out to be made of tin.

You are your own man and can choose to speak when and where you please. The telephone need no longer thrust a lance of ice into your guts. You no longer have to take part in meetings, justify yourself and your work, or go to large parties. Nobody is going to ask you to do the impossible. If you don't wish to talk you don't. You can sit on your porch, smoke a pipe, and look at your fields.

As the pressures ease, so the speech gets better. You still stutter, but it is no longer a fight to speak. You can choose your own verbal battle-grounds.

Although I am hardly in the first bloom of youth, the young person I used to be still lives within me and looks out at the world through my eyes. I don't consider myself old. Nevertheless, when I took early retirement to be my own master the relief was tremendous. The tensions of anticipating the talking involved in getting through an ordinary working day were greater than I realized at the time. After I left, my speech improved rapidly.

Since then I foolishly became involved in high-pressure talking from time to time, and the tensions built up again. After a week or so the speech began to fracture. I have learned to take the pressures off my speech and enjoy my fluency.

The way a stutter affects you in old age depends, of course, on what kind of person you are. If your stuttering has defeated you throughout your life and driven you into unhappy solitude, you will look back sadly with many regrets and still feel the pain of old emotional wounds that never heal. One of the saddest pictures I ever saw was an illustration of what the caption called 'An Old Stutterer' in one of the textbooks. He was well dressed, but the despair in his eyes and the tired, sagging features went straight to the heart. He had been utterly crushed by his stutter and society's cruelty.

I have met very few older stutterers who have been so totally defeated. Most of them are more like old soldiers, taking it easy after battle, with the pain of their honourable scars well under control. There may be some who look back with bitterness and wish that their lives could have been different unhindered by the ball and chain of disfluency, but the general feeling seems to be that life has been good and full of challenges and richness. Without the stutter they wouldn't have become the people they are. It has moulded them from infancy.

NINE

The road ahead

'Yesterday is not ours to recover,
but tomorrow is ours to win or lose.'

Anonymous

A stuttering friend who was a born pessimist was also something of a blues singer. During World War II, he was sure that he was going to get the chop, and used to sit in the cold, damp Nissen hut strumming a tinny old banjo and singing a mournful little song:

'Ah went up on this mountain,
Saw as far as ah could see,
Ah went up on this mountain
'N the blues had me.'

He always sang the same verse from the same song. It was our only music apart from a rickety spring-driven turntable and a scarred old record of the Anvil Chorus, so we put up with it. He was wrong. He survived. As far as I know he's still wailing his pessimistic little dirge.

The great thing about people who stutter is that, unlike my woeful friend, so many of them are optimists. When one type of therapy fails, they try another, and then another. Hoping, always hoping. They may fall flat on their faces and make fools of themselves, but they pick themselves up and try a new tack against the headwinds of life. Give them a chance and they'll grab it and run with it.

What have people who stutter to look forward to in a world that has produced so many technical marvels but remains in such a state of political, economic and moral chaos? Will scientists soon find out what causes a child to start stuttering? Will somebody find a real cure? Will the new technology make life easier for the severely disfluent? Will society learn to accept people with speech and other disabilities more readily? Will the partially disabled have a louder voice in dealing with legal and bureaucratic injustices and prejudices? The answers to these questions will determine the future happiness and social effectiveness of millions of stutterers and other disabled people.

Technology is one of the things man does best, so it is fair to assume that there will be considerable advances in speech technology in the next twenty-five years, provided that governments allocate sufficient research support. The science of psychology and neurology are gradually unravelling the mysteries of the brain's processes and how they affect our behaviour, and the old qualitative type of psychology is giving way to a new science based on firmer neurological and biochemical foundations.

People who contend that stuttering is just learned behaviour may ask, 'Why bother about all this research? Why not treat the symptom?' Several intractable complaints – including depression, schizophrenia, malaria, poliomyelitis, tuberculosis, and smallpox – yielded to treatment once their causes were understood. Fifty years from now we shall probably look back on today's speech therapy as groping in the dark, which is how we have come to regard the older methods of relaxation and rhythmics.

Conditioning methods like fluency shaping therapy and combinations of speech rehabilitation and psychotherapy get better every year and will continue to do so unless therapists polarize into fluency shapers and stuttering modifiers. The more fanatical proponents of fluency shaping tend to look down their noses at the complex, personal approach of stuttering modifiers, and some of the latter have a hunch that the human brain has its own ideas about how far it can be conditioned. It is hoped that the clinicians will bring the best in both approaches to bear on the problem. When we understand the functions of the brain better, particularly the role of neurotransmitters at the nerves' synapses, and find out to what extent the ear is involved in the mechanics of speech, treatment will develop on a firmer basis.

There is no real barrier to finding out whether or not stuttering or the inclination to stutter is encoded in our genes. The information could be obtained from studies of twins and siblings living with natural and adoptive parents, by calculating the frequencies of stuttering in all these groups. This type of study has yielded important insights into schizophrenia. All it needs is the will, the time, and the money.

If stuttering proves to be genetically mediated this does not mean that nothing can be done about the disability. Each gene produces compounds that trigger psysiological processes. When the processes are understood, their abnormalities may respond to treatment. (Again, schizophrenia and other disorders mediated by neurotransmitters and enzyme systems come to mind.) Knowledge about the genetic basis of stuttering could provide an early warning system and enable children to be treated earlier.

A stutterer reading the literature about his problem comes across a few points that strike sparks of relevance in his mind. Some of the sparks fade as he reads further, but others continue to glow and illuminate the whole stuttering scene. A few of the points are old ones that have tarnished with time; they deserve polishing again in view of new knowledge. Good examples are laterality and its relationship to stuttering and the old organic idea of bugs in the brain's computer. Other points are more innovative – for example, the question of whether excessive anxiety about speech is encoded in our genes or associated with malfunctions in the areas of the brain concerned with our emotions. A reconsideration of the role of the middle-ear muscles in speech also raises glimmers of understanding and even of hope. Novel approaches to operant conditioning using biofeedback have great promise in treating anxiety-mediated disabilities like stuttering.

Laterality revisited

The cerebral dominance theory suggested that the left side of the brain's cerebral cortex, where the speech centres are usually located, must dominate the right side in order to time correctly the nerve impulses from the brain's motor centre to the muscles of the lips, tongue, and jaw and enable a person to speak normally. It was suggested that stuttering could be caused by a lack of dominance of the side of the brain dealing with speech. Many speech therapists clung to this neurological straw for decades, but the idea fell into disrepute. The results of recent research indicate that the theory is worthy of re-examination.

The ability to speak is relatively new in the evolutionary time scale, and speech is possible because man has two unique speech centres in the brain that enable him to put ideas into words. These centres are Broca's and Wernicke's areas.

Broca's area is on the left side of the brain a little above and to the front of the tip of the ear in most normal right-handed people. It is responsible for programming the mechanics of speech. Broca's area controls the motor cortex, a strip of specialized tissue arching over the brain from ear to ear like a headphone, which activates the muscles involved in speech and other movements. When Broca's area is damaged the speech is understandable but ungrammatical, slow, and hesitant. Verbs, pronouns, and connecting words like prepositions are left out. A typical sentence would be 'Church Sunday eleven o'clock sermon.' Damage to this area affects writing in a similar way.

Wernicke's area is concerned with language and plays a major role in speaking, comprehension of written and spoken words, and sentence construction. When this area is damaged the words may be spoken clearly and fluently with perfect grammar but make no sense at all.

Investigations of these brain areas have indicated that what someone is going to say is organized in Wernicke's area. If the word is read optically it travels from the eye to the visual area at the back of the brain and then to Wernicke's area along a nerve bundle – the 'angular gyrus.' If the word is heard, the signal travels from the brain's auditory area a little to the front of Wernicke's area and then onwards to the latter.

Wernicke's area is both a junction box and a signal processor. After it processes the signals, they pass on to Broca's area, which produces a detailed, co-ordinated program for speech and flashes messages to the nearby motor cortex, which in turn activates the articulatory muscles. All the nerve tissues, together with their linkages, need to be in working order for a person to say, 'Good morning. I would like three litres please,' to the milkman.

This simple model of speech tends to get a little scrambled when left- and right-handedness enter the picture, since it is now known that differences in handedness are associated with different positions of the speech centres in the brain. About 99 per cent, or more, of normal, right-handed people have their speech and language centres (Broca's and Wernicke's areas) on the left side of the brain. Their brain's right side is more concerned with matters of space, time, seeing things as a whole, and intuition. Some people's brains have a limited capability for language on the right side, but in right-handed people most of the language business is carried out on the left side. If the right-handed person writes with his right hand so that the nib points toward him, he may have his language centres on the opposite side of the brain – the right side. The reversed-pen stance is uncommon in right-handers, accounting for only about 1 per cent. By contrast to most right-handers, some left-handed people have their speech centres on the right side of the brain and the space-time-intuition function on the left. However, if the left-handed person writes with his left hand in such a way that the pen's nib points toward him, his speech centres tend to be on the left side, as with most right-handers. Eye movements and writing position reveal a great deal about the workings of the brain, and Dr Jerre Levy of the University of Chicago used this fact in her elegant experiments on brain laterality and asymmetry.[1]

An experiment to test whether stuttering is more common in people with the speech centres on the right side of the cerebral cortex than in those with speech centres on the left side would produce useful insights into whether stuttering is associated with reversed, abnormal brain circuitry. The implied complication of a reversal of speech centres in relation to the brain's visual and auditory centres and the motor cortex makes the mind reel.

My own case is complicated because I am partly ambidextrous. I throw with my right hand and do precision work with my left. I get on a bicycle on the right side and, in my riding days, I would have preferred to have mounted my horses from the right side, but they violently objected. I use my left hand for many tasks, but kick a football in the wrong direction with the right foot. The real tangle in the wool is that I write from left to right with my right hand, and scribble from right to left with my left hand, always with the pen's nib away from me. I can even, with a little practice, write with both hands at once, one script a mirror image of the other. I am in good company, because Leonardo da Vinci could do the same; he wrote all his notes with his left hand in mirror script. If my speech centres are associated with my handedness, I am not at all sure where they are located and just hope that I have Broca's and Wernicke's speech and language areas in the ordinary place, on the left side.

It is interesting that two of my daughters write with their left hands, and their pens' nibs point away from them, making it remotely possible that their speech centres are on the right side of the brain instead of the usual left. Neither of them stutters.

If stuttering proves to be associated with displacement of the speech centres or abnormal cerebral dominance and this appears to be one of the tributaries feeding the stutter's main stream, at least therapists will know what they are dealing with and can decide where to focus their attention.

The brain's neural network

Whenever I am accused by my wife of having a lot of nerve, I exasperate her by nodding in agreement, reminding her that I have about 10^{11} (or about 100,000 million) neurons or nerve cells with about 10^{15} (1,000 million million) nerve contacts – the synapses – in addition to billions of interlaced, short, thread-like fibres (dendrites) between the neurons.[2] The long fibres (axons) of the neuron cells are the main wires of the circuit, and each one has its own protective insulation – the fatty myelin sheath. A typical neuron may have 1,000 to 10,000 synaptic connections and receive information from 1,000 or more other neurons. The sheer number of units and connections in the circuitry is staggering, and the brain makes our most advanced computers look primitive by comparison.

This complex machine works by biochemical processes and electrical impulses. The neuron's chemistry sends an electrical impulse along the axon to a club-like junction (the synapse), which is connected to a receiving neuron. The two are not strictly connected, because there is a minute space between the receiver neuron and the receptive synaptic swelling. The swollen synapse stores a chemical transmitter (neurotransmitter), which is released into the small gap by the nerve's electrical impulse and changes the electrical state of the receptor neuron, which may fire and send its message, or not, depending on its function. If the chemical transmitter of the synapse does not work properly, the circuit misfires and the next neuron cannot pass on its electrical message. When the neuron's electrical discharges are out of synchronization, or the axons are damaged, the electrical circuits break down and we have problems.[3]

Fortunately, the brain can repair itself to some extent, so that people can function quite well after certain kinds of brain damage, although in some instances even minor injury can have devastating effects. It depends on where the problem lies and on the age of the individual.

When a person has a stroke, and the nerves that control the movements of muscles involved in speech (Broca's area) are damaged, the victim speaks poorly, although he can still sing with ease. This parallels the plight of people who stutter severely but can also sing. Damage to Wernicke's area results in fluent, grammatical nonsensical speech.

Damage to the speech areas does not necessarily mean that the speech will be out of action for ever. While it is true that Broca's and Wernicke's areas play a major role in speech and language, other areas of the brain can take over their functions to some extent. For example, a person with his main speech centres on the left side of the brain may have a limited speech capability on his right side that can help to some extent in a crisis. The damaged brain tissue cannot recover, but neurons near the damaged site may take over.[4]

If the zone damaged in Broca's area is small, the chances of partial recovery are quite good.[5] Children, in particular, recover remarkably well; and, curiously, left-handed people recover better than right-handers – laterality rears its puzzling head again. Moreover, a stroke victim with damage on the left side of his brain is often depressed about his disability, while patients with damage on the right side are often unconcerned about their predicament.[6] Speech disruption caused by lesions in the speech areas on the left side of the brain are likely to be associated with anxiety.

These are facts, but at this point it is necessary to wade into a swamp of speculation. Consider the case of a child who is slightly more disfluent than usual. In the absence of bad therapy, stress, penalties, and ridicule there is a good chance that the disfluency will disappear in later childhood, although this depends upon the severity of the stuttering. If the child is penalized, stressed, rejected, and ridiculed, he will be anxious about his speech, and it is likely that his stuttering will get worse and tend to reinforce itself. However, even when his speech is bad, he will be able to sing fluently most of the time.

The key points are that the child is disfluent but can sing, often recovers, and may be anxious. The question is whether this picture fits the template of a person with a left-side (speech-zone) abnormality of the brain in, for example, Broca's area. The answer is not exactly, but there are a few points of contact. If a left-side speech zone of a stutterer's brain were damaged or abnormal, neighbouring neurons or some other brain zone could in time take over some of the speech function, and the quality of the speech would depend upon the degree of damage. If this were the case, many children would recover – and, in fact, many stuttering children spontaneously lose their stutters. Many patients with damage in Broca's area can sing. Anxiety about the disability would be expected with left-side brain damage, and stutterers' anxiety about their speech is well known.

The behaviour of left-side stroke victims with damage in Broca's area will strike echoes in many stutterers' minds, and there is a little evidence of brain abnormality in the language areas of dyslexics' brains. There is a need to reconsider the question of whether organic abnormalities in the brain affect the onset of stuttering and to examine the possibility of left-side abnormalities in the speech areas in the light of evidence from stroke victims and dyslexics. Recent research is moving along these lines.

My wife and I knew a very old lady in England who liked to sit in her sunny room, look at the flowers, and cheerfully chat to visitors. When she was younger she was very articulate and talkative, and her friends described her as loving but fierce. Her speech centres or their connections had deteriorated in her old age, and she found it difficult to speak. Her speech was not the laboured articulation and telegraphic syntax of a person with damage in Broca's area, nor was it the fluent, grammatical, but nonsensical speech of a person damaged in Wernicke's area. She certainly wasn't a clutterer. When she spoke she made sense, but she repeated sounds and went into severe blocks of five seconds or more, just like a stutterer.

As we sat and talked to this fascinating woman we were both struck by the similarity of her speech to that of an adult stutterer, the only difference being her freedom from anxiety.

Experts will probably say that her so-called stutter was not a real stutter, but something like it. Nevertheless, except for her lack of fear, her speech fitted the stuttering pattern exactly. As I listened I heard a carbon copy of my own speech. The old lady was almost completely deaf, and the complications of anxiety and hearing were absent, so it seems that speech patterns very similar to stuttering can develop from deterioration of the tissues in the brain's speech areas. It is unwise to conclude from this that stuttering is simply due to brain abnormality, but it suggests that the possible association between brain structure and stuttering is worthy of close examination.

Understanding anxiety

It is not known whether a child's stuttering stems from anxiety or whether the anxiety is caused by the stuttering, but there is little doubt that anxiety contributes a great deal to the growth and consolidation of stuttering behaviour. It is fair to ask, therefore, whether better methods will be developed to understand and deal with this anxiety.

The obvious way to reduce a stutterer's anxiety is to

remove, reduce, or control his stutter, and this underlies the fact that increased fluency increases fluency. The stuttering modification therapy of the Iowa school focuses on these fears and tries to dispel them by teaching the stutterer to adopt realistic, objective attitudes and to *feel* his fluency. Many patients with severe stutters like mine can still be overwhelmed by unexpected fears about particular words even after years of therapy, to the extent that at times it seems like a phobia about speaking. If this so-called phobia has been learned, it can be unlearned – unless it is caused by an inheritance of excessive fearfulness about communicating. It must be remembered that a stutterer's fear of stuttering may be an appropriate response to disfluency, since society takes such exception to it. Nevertheless, the degree of anxiety may be abnormal.

There is evidence that excessive fearfulness can be inherited. The basenjis mentioned earlier inherited a fearful response to man, and laboratory rats were found to have distinctive genetic strains quite different in their fearfulness (reactivity), one strain being ten times more fearful than the other. Furthermore, hybridizing fearful and less fearful rats produces rats with intermediate behaviour, so genes seem to be involved. Animals inherit specific fears (e.g., of objects looming over them), as well as fears of many things that threaten their survival.[7]

Anxiety can be learned in infancy. At a very early age a child will respond fearfully when what he sees or hears does not match his previous experience. Although the relationship of fear to cognitive mismatch is complex,[8] it raises the question of whether a small child used to a fluent mother most of the day could be alarmed by hearing a disfluent, stuttering father communicating in a way that does not match the child's experience and expectation. There is some evidence that a child with a stuttering mother is more likely to develop a stutter than otherwise.

The possibility that abnormalities in the brain's nerve network cause excessive anxiety must be considered, but the chemical relationships between the different parts of the brain are so complex that it is hard to get a clear picture. In *The Tangled Wing*, Melvin Konner makes clear that abnormalities in the balance between the components of our centres mediating emotion (in the limbic system) and damage to the insulating myelin sheaths of the message-carrying axons could produce inappropriate or excessively fearful responses.[9] Nevertheless, much more information is needed before the biochemical and biological nature of fear is understood and before anxiety can be treated with confidence.

Several drugs can be used to treat anxiety. Valium (Diazepam) is a good example. This drug influences the release of a chemical neurotransmitter (gamma-aminobutyric acid) at synaptic junctions of message-carrying axon fibres in the brain. Unfortunately, although Valium reduces anxiety it also decreases alertness.[10] Alcohol affects the chemical signals of the nerves and reduces anxiety in a similar way to Valium, which is doubtless the reason why alcohol is so popular in our fearful world. Anxiety can be modified by drugs, but at the price of side effects many patients are reluctant to pay. Doubtless better drugs will evolve. Cimetidine, for example, is sometimes used instead of Valium, but all drugs are likely to have side effects.

Attempts have been made to treat some phobias by brain surgery, but it is to be hoped that this is not attempted with stutterers until more is known about the neurology of speech, and of fear, and about whether the anxiety of stutterers is a cause or an effect or both. The memory of tongue-butchering Dr Dieffenbach is still too fresh in many stutterers' memories.

For the time being, therefore, it seems appropriate for scientists to try to probe the role of anxiety in stuttering and for speech therapists to try to control the fears by conventional therapy (possibly assisted by better psychotherapy and carefully administered drugs), while realizing that excessive anxiety is only part of the complex stuttering syndrome.

I never cease to feel a sense of awe that I carry around with me an incredibly complex and efficient organic computer protected by my thick skull. The brain is *me*, and from it I look out upon the world and flash signals along my axons, relay the signals across the synaptic gaps, and activate my sight centres at the back of the brain that allow me to see. If I want to talk about what I see, signals are flashed to my language centre, which alerts Broca's area, which in turn signals the neurons that control my lip, tongue, and jaw muscles and make my larynx vibrate. All in a flash. As I see something else, new signals are generated and new words are spoken.

Every thought we have, every movement we make, and every emotion we feel are the result of billions of flashing electrochemical signals, sorted, co-ordinated, and monitored in the soft tissues of our brain. When I was a foetus my neural network miraculously grew from a few cells, the neurons' axons weaving their way in my brain tissues, nudged and coaxed by biochemical compounds to make the right connections with other brain cells. When the wrong connections were made they often aborted so that better connections could be made. Even after I was born, the slender, branched dendrites growing out from the nerve cells continued to grow, each new experience adding new branches.

It is amazing that most people get their brain circuits wired up more or less in the right way. The probability that something will go wrong as the network develops under the guidance of the biochemical stew generated by both our genes and our environment seems very high. Nature must be forgiven if she occasionally makes a mistake.

Sound and speech

In 1974 Ronald L. Webster of Hollins College, Virginia, said that investigation of the role of the middle-ear muscles was 'the most meaningful potential direction for the conduct of future research on the problem of stuttering.'[11] There is a wealth of evidence that delayed feedback of the sound of a person's speech can cause disfluency and that masking the feedback completely can make a stutterer fluent, so it is likely that the ear is involved in the act of speaking.

The middle-ear (tympanum) involves two small muscles (the tensor tympani and the stapedius) attached to three small movable bones – the hammer (malleus), the anvil (incus), and the stirrup (stapes). These bones form a lever that picks up the sound vibrations from the ear-drum, amplifies them, and relays them to an inner membrane, which vibrates and enables us to hear. The tensor tympani muscle, attached to the malleus, dampens loud noises and protects the fragile eardrum. It is activated by a nerve with a delay of about 150 milliseconds. The stapedius muscle, which shields the inner ear from an excessive amount of relayed sound, is attached to the stapes and responds in about 60 milliseconds. These two muscles also hold the three bones of the chain in position, and contract not only in response to sound but also about 65 to 100 milliseconds before a person speaks. The muscle contraction appears to be part of an involuntary preparation for the act of speaking. The middle-ear muscles seem to be involved in speech both in stutterers and in fluent speakers.

A study of the movements of the muscles of the middle ear of five stutterers indicated that the contractions occurred at the time of stuttering. However, when the stutterers spoke fluently, the muscles contracted in the normal way, just before speaking.[12] The timing of the ear's muscle contractions associated with stuttering may be abnormal. Caution is necessary in interpreting this fact, since a stutterer's tension can produce many abnormal physiological and muscle responses. Nevertheless, one stutterer who had the middle-ear muscles removed during an operation for some other disorder found that his stutter decreased from about 8–12 per cent disfluency to 1–3 per cent, and the improvement persisted even though he still had intact the middle-ear muscles in the other ear. His hearing was slightly reduced, but this was dealt with by a hearing aid.[13]

It seems possible, therefore, that the contractions of the ear muscles of stutterers may be erratic or out of phase and may disrupt auditory feedback to such an extent that they interfere with speaking. Whether the pre-speech ear-muscle contraction is vital to speech initiation remains to be seen. If this proves to be the case, it may lead to new treatment opportunities. However, some scientists feel that this middle-ear theory is a backwater rather than in the mainstream of current research.

It seems clear that sound and hearing are much more involved in speech than was previously thought, and that speech may be guided (or misguided) by specific auditory cues. Unfortunately, we still don't know how speech and hearing interact, and the operation on the stutterer's ear was a one-shot affair, so we are not likely to see people with stutters lining up to get the tiny muscles chopped out of their middle ears.

Biofeedback

These days it is very fashionable to sit with small circular electrodes attached to the muscles of your forehead listening to a biofeedback beeper signal that you have managed to persuade yourself to relax. When I worked in a city I used to survey people's foreheads for the hickies left by the tacky kisses of the biofeedback electrodes. There were more than you'd think.

The principles of biofeedback are not new. Any mental and physical activity causes changes in the body's electrochemistry. Tensed muscles send out different electrical signals than relaxed muscles; some forms of mental activity send out different electrical brain waves than others; and many processes modify our body temperature. If these signals can be measured and amplified into indicators a person can see, hear, or feel, then theoretically he can control the bodily activities that generate the signals by thinking in a passive way or by deliberately creating particular inner feelings.

Although this sounds like witchcraft, most people have at one time or another controlled their bodies with their minds to reduce anxiety, discomfort, or severe pain. On many of the occasions when I've shivered with cold I've thought warm thoughts and felt much better. People in great agony can sometimes consciously ride with the pain and convince themselves it is receding. When parents tell their children that they can do almost anything if they put their minds to it, they are not far wrong as far as the body's functions are concerned.

The most commonly measured signals of the body are temperature, muscle tension (EMG biofeedback), and alpha waves from the brain (EEG biofeedback). The last two are most relevant to stuttering.

Electromyographic (EMG) feedback has been used with some success to treat a wide range of disorders. Barbara B. Brown, in *Stress and the Art of Biofeedback*,[14] lists twelve emotional problems (including anxiety, phobias, tension headaches, insomnia, and depression), five psychosomatic problems (including asthma, hypertension, and intestinal disorders), and ten physical problems (including painful muscle spasms, spasticity, cerebral palsy, and migraines) that have responded to EMG biofeedback. Anxiety is particularly responsive to the technique, which consequently has promise as a treatment for stuttering.

For several days I sat plugged into a biofeedback machine having great fun making the monitor bleep to my changes in muscle tension. I became so good at it that I could play games and perplexed the therapist by bouncing around the readings just by thinking and feeling in different ways. I was a natural feedback patient and could relax myself into a near-trance while I spoke fluently. The trouble was that my control over my state of relaxation disappeared as soon as I walked out of the clinic.

I still feel that the biofeedback method can play a useful role in speech therapy. The assertion that felt fluency helps to keep you fluent is true, but some stutterers have never felt what it is like to speak fluently in a relaxed manner in public. It feels wonderful. You try and remember what the feeling felt like, but it's very difficult to measure, monitor, and use on demand.

EMG was tested by Guitar in his laboratory, using electrodes on the larynx, chin, upper lip, and the forehead's frontalis muscle. The electrical activity was amplified into a humming tone. Three patients tried to keep the tone as low as possible, and when the lowest level was achieved they read sentences that included difficult words. Similar trials were run without the feedback. In all cases the EMG biofeedback reduced stuttering, and the improvement persisted for several months, even with telephone calls.[15] Whether the muscle relaxation helped the speech, or the humming tone provided some form of distraction are points in question. Oliver Bloodstein commented that EMG feedback seems well suited to eliminate the excessive tension of stutterers and that it holds considerable promise.[16] Other scientists have studied the use of EMG biofeedback to treat stuttering, but the technique is still in its infancy.

Alpha-wave feedback is concerned with the variations of the alpha rhythms (9 to 12 Hz) from a person's brain. There are several types of brain waves, but high alpha activity is associated with a state of relaxed wakefulness and receptivity. This technique, also in its infancy, consists of attaching the EEG electrodes to the scalp so that the patient can learn to control his alpha waves by observing them on the screen and passively modifying them. Although there is often a great deal of interference with the waves, the method has helped many people with tension problems. In Texas, hyperactive children with stuttering and insomnia are said to have responded well to alpha-wave training.[17] If biofeedback can help stutterers to control their anxiety about speaking it may prove to be one of the more useful modern tools.

New information will provide fresh insights into the causes and treatment of stuttering, but more funds are needed to support research. People who stutter should make their collective, hesitant voices heard in high places and clamour for more attention to their problems. Ingenious man should be able to come up with a few answers after two thousand years of research on tangled tongues.

The information age

The world is changing rapidly, and stutterers, like other people, will need to adapt if they are to survive. The rapidly increasing world population, the spread of mechanization, and the scarcity of natural resources are likely to increase competition for food, homes, and jobs. These stresses will place more pressure on a stutterer's speech and may increase people's impatience with the disfluent and other handicapped. Technology is advancing more rapidly than our social values. If we make mistakes we can make them faster and more often. People who stutter will need all their resourcefulness to survive.

If we can believe the futurists, we are entering the Information Age, where communication will be paramount. A person with a stutter will find that some of the new technology will help him; but some situations may prove hard to handle.

Computers are here to be used and misused whether we like it or not. They have invaded our homes and schools, and communication by video screen and computer print-out will soon become commonplace. A stutterer could find that he needs to speak less. You don't have to be fluent to punch keys, look at screens, and read messages on pieces of paper.

People using computers tend to lean heavily on pure logic both at home and in the workplace. They tend to use the areas of the brain devoted to logic more than those from which derive the 'human' attributes of holistic thinking, intuition, compassion, and love. Logic can be so powerful and convincing that people tend to discount their better selves when convinced by cold figures. The brutalities of the slave trade were justified by the cold logic of economics and the quest for power. Humanity is left out of too many equations.

If the use of computers results in a coldly 'rational' society, handicapped people are in for a bad time. Fortunately computers can, when used as extensions to the mind rather than as minds themselves, process data very rapidly. They provide access to huge amounts of information, and this could be of enormous benefit in studies of stuttering. Complex, interactive computer models of businesses, forest ecosystems, and physiological processes have been constructed and work well in their own fields. All of these systems, like a stutter, involve many interacting factors. Perhaps one day a computer model of a stutter can be created and manipulated to discover better methods of treatment.

When I heard about electronic conferencing, mail, and noticeboards my heart sang at the thought of the imminent demise of my arch enemy, the oral telephone. I ran to the nearest computer store where some bright fellow plugged a modem into our computer and unplugged a great many dollars from our bank account. We were all set to Communicate.

The modem is called a Smart Modem because it is clever enough to operate in two gears, 300 bauds and 1,200 bauds, slow and fast. The problem was that I was not as smart as the modem, and the massive instruction manual defeated me. A colleague who kindly offered to advise left a gaggle of commands flying around my empty head, each of which escaped through one ear or the other in a very short time. I tried. I even achieved buzzing and clicking noises, but no messages. I was, however, entirely successful in promoting the cash flow of the telephone company. In two days of practice I ran up a $70 telephone bill.

So my modem with all its baudy potential sits on my desk, and the thick manual stands unsullied on the bookshelf beside my other tattered computer manuals. Back we went to the bosoms of old Ma Bell's merry band of telephone operators.

In spite of my dim-witted disappointment, electronic conferencing could help people who stutter if they and their colleagues have the wherewithal to buy the hardware, the type of minds that can understand computerese, and the cash flow to keep paying the telephone bills.

If a stutterer takes the trouble to become computer literate, many new job avenues will be available to him where his disfluency will not be a major handicap. The Information Age could benefit the disfluent and other disabled considerably if they have the courage to plunge into this new world.

The silent minority: not so minor

In times of economic crisis the political economists look hungrily at the funds allocated to hospitals, schools, universities, pensions, and programs for the handicapped. Soon after any election, the headlines appear in the press: 'Plans to Cut Social Services.' This is perplexing, since most people are under the impression that politicians are elected to serve society.

Fortunately, the electorate can do something about it. The handicapped have a more powerful lobby than they realize. Quite apart from obvious, severe disabilities, there are many that are partial or periodic but nevertheless disabling. About 1 per cent of people stutter; about 1 per cent are dyslexic; 1 per cent have schizophrenia; and many more have agoraphobia, severe sight or hearing disabilities, and damage to the brain's speech centres by ruptured aneurysms or cerebral embolisms. If someone took the trouble to calculate the numbers of people disabled to the extent that it interferes with their ability to work unaided and to participate effectively in society, the so-called disabled minority would turn out to be not so minor after all.

Without taking into account the elderly, at least 6 per cent of the population have functional disabilities of one kind or another. In North America alone there must be fifteen million disabled people who can vote or will vote in the future. This would be doubled if the disabled old people were taken into account, and doubled again if the parents, siblings, husbands, wives, and friends of the disabled were included. A total of about sixty million people could have a loud voice in the policies of the nations of North America if they made the effort.

There is increasing evidence of militancy among the old and the disabled. The elderly have appeared on the streets waving banners protesting reductions in pensions, facilities, and rights. Unfortunately, their voices have not been loud enough. They can't go on strike and they haven't the money to take cases to court. Their efforts are dissipated. The only way disabled people can be heard is to act in a large group to get political clout. This shouldn't be necessary, but we don't live in Shangri-La.

Charters of human rights of one kind or another exist in many countries. The people who seem to benefit most from these rights are criminals and other public nuisances who howl 'Discrimination!' when they feel the hand of retribution on their shoulders. Nevertheless, the mechanisms for the disabled to assert their rights are there to be used. We should learn how to use them. There is no need to put up with blatant maltreatment and discrimination. Every few years the voters can elect men of conscience into positions of power – if they can find them.

Shifting attitudes: the quiet revolution

In spite of the materialism of the world's developed countries, there has been a quiet revolution in people's attitudes since 1950. Old values have been reconsidered and rejected, accepted, or modified. Gross exploitation of natural resources regardless of its effect on the environment is no longer accepted as unavoidable; progress is no longer measured just by economic growth; some economists include values other than dollars in their calculations of costs and benefits; women are less frequently regarded as second-class citizens; and efforts are being made to secure the rights of all people, regardless of race, sex, age, creed, or colour. Many citizens have opted out of the race for power, possessions, and money to live simpler, more satisfying lives and are attempting to raise their children to share their values. The 'Back to Basics' movement at times became a little too basic, but the idea of re-evaluation is both welcome and refreshing.

The growth of new religious sects and the popularity of evangelists, both good and bad, suggest that people are looking for new sets of values (or new ways of looking at old values) and are prepared to spend time, money, and energy on consolidating and spreading their new beliefs. Certainly, the barbarians are still with us. Predators still prey on the weak and defenceless, but the growth of grass-roots movements to think and do things in better ways is encouraging. People of goodwill and conscience have votes. The old walls of established and outmoded attitudes can be cracked.

Society's attitudes toward the disabled are immeasurably better than they were fifty years ago. I have clear, childhood memories of destitute amputees in the 1930s pushing themselves around on low wooden trolleys and begging for pennies; and of processions of jeering children following severely disabled spastics down the street. Hunchbacks were fair game for gangs of youths out for an evening's mischief, and albinos and individuals with harelips or cleft palates were openly ridiculed. Today these brutalities are much less open and less frequent. Most of today's discrimination is indirect, hidden, or unintentional.

During the 1940s, my wife, Joan, went to a girls' school in England where good manners were high on the list of priorities. On one occasion a teacher said to Joan, 'What would you do if you met a person in a wheelchair or someone who was severely deformed? You wouldn't turn away would you?' The implication was that, whatever your fears, you treated the disabled like anyone else, with courtesy and consideration. Other ways of behaving were just not imaginable. She was not ordered to behave in a particular way, but was shown that there was no other acceptable course of action. She and the teacher took it for granted.

Society has basic standards of behaviour that include honesty, truthfulness, and finding non-violent solutions for problems. Laws exist to see that these standards are enforced. In general only major infringements of law reach the courts, and it is impossible to legislate to outlaw minor dishonesties, lies, and acts of aggression. You could fill the bookshelves with legislation to deal with injustices and discrimination, but no amount of legislation will compel people to cease their rudeness, rejection, and insensitivity when they meet the disabled unless they want to. It is necessary, therefore, to 'raise society's consciousness' about such matters.

Most people are willing to listen, learn, and change their attitudes when they know the facts. If stutterers are to live without the glass wall between themselves and society, they must make sure that the facts reach the public. School is the obvious place to start, but the radio, press, and television offer tremendous opportunities for informing and influencing the public. It will take time, but society's attitudes toward people with tangled tongues can be changed for the better without punitive, unenforceable legislation. Stutterers and their families and friends, as well as the various speech associations, could have a tremendous impact on the public through the media if they were to make the effort.

The outlook for changing society's behaviour toward the disfluent is promising, but it won't just happen on its own.

Conclusion

This book has been a long journey. During its writing I resurrected old memories, some painful, some warm, some funny. Like any other journey, it was an education, and assembling the information gave me new insights into my speech. At times I walked on dangerous ground. Some of the chapters caused my speech to deteriorate temporarily, and at times it was hard to write objectively, but I was sustained by the memory of the warmth and courage of all the hundreds of stuttering children, adolescents, and adults I have met, and of the dedicated therapists with whom I worked. And how we worked!

People who stutter deserve better from society, and maybe this book will help in a small way to achieve this. I still find it an effort to speak, but can look back over fifty-five years of hesitant, unpredictable speech and more than fifty years of therapy not with regret, but with a sense of quiet jubilation that I have met so many wonderful people, lived such a rich life, and encountered so many challenges. I have seen the darkest and the brightest sides of humanity, and the bright side reigns supreme.

Notes

The abbreviation *JSHD* used in these notes refers to the *Journal of Speech and Hearing Disorders*.

1 Many therapists are sceptical about the use of the Edinburgh Masker and deplore excessive claims in the media about its usefulness. Other therapists recognize the value of the masker for some stutterers, particularly those who have impediments that have not responded well to treatment. The incident described in this Preface explains how it worked for me on a particular occasion. This does not imply that it is the answer to all stuttering. The masker is discussed later in the book in more detail.

2 Although 'stammering' is the present Old World term for the New World's 'stuttering,' the term 'stut' has a long and honourable pedigree. In 1627, Sir Francis Bacon, the scientist, philosopher, and man of letters, wrote in *Sylva Sylvarum*: 'Divers, we see, doe Stut. The Cause may be ... the Refrigeration of the Tongue; Whereby it is lesse apt to move ...; And we see that those that Stut, if they drinke Wine moderately, they Stut less, because it heateth ... it may be (though rarely) the Driness of the Tongue which maketh it lesse apt to move, as well as Cold; For it is an Affect that it cometh to some Wise and Great Men; as it did unto Moses, who was *Linguae Praepiditae*.'

Bacon's suggestion that stuttering was caused by the coldness or dryness of the tongue perpetuated a myth originating in the teachings of Aristotle and Hippocrates. The term 'stammering' was used by Benjamin Alexander, MD, as early as 1769 in his translation of Morgagni's *Treatise on Stuttering*.

3 A great many terms, many of them poorly defined, were used for 'stuttering' in the early literature. Hippocrates' *'trauloi'* seems to refer to speech defects in general, but Aristotle's *'ischnophonoi'* was used specifically for stuttering. Stuttering and cluttering were

grouped under the title of *'psellismus'* in the seventeenth century. *'Balbus,' 'balbuties,'* and *'batarismus'* were used for stuttering, but the usage tended to be erratic. Stuttering in early times is described in some detail by R.W. Rieber and J. Wollock in 'The historical roots of the theory and therapy of stuttering,' in R.W. Rieber, ed., *The Problem of Stuttering* (New York: Elsevier 1977).

4 'Cluttering' is best described as a disability consisting of rapid, jerky, slurred, jumbled speech, with words repeated or left out. The words come in rapid spurts. Most clutterers can speak fluently when they speak slowly and carefully, which is not necessarily true of people who stutter severely.

CHAPTER 1

1 United States Department of Health and Human Services, *Stuttering: Hope through Research* (Washington, DC: National Institute of Health, Publication 81–2250, 1981)

CHAPTER 2

1 A. Mehrabian, 'Nonverbal communication,' *Nebraska Symposium on Communication* (Lincoln, Neb.: Nebraska University Press 1972); and R.P. Harrison, 'Nonverbal behavior: an approach to human communication,' in R.W. Budd and B.D. Ruben, eds., *Approaches to Human Communication* (Rochelle Park, NJ: Spartan Books 1972), 253–68

2 J. Fast, *Body Language* (New York: Pocket Books 1975); D. Morris, *Man Watching: A Field Guide to Human Behavior* (New York: Abrams 1977); Harrison, 'Nonverbal behavior'

3 O. Bloodstein, *A Handbook on Stuttering*, 3rd ed. (Chicago, Ill.: National Easter Seals Society 1981), 87, 99

4 Ibid., 80; and W. Johnson and associates, *The Onset of Stuttering* (Minneapolis, Minn.: University of Minnesota Press 1959)

5 Bloodstein, *Handbook on Stuttering*, 3rd ed., 160–1

6 J.O. Graf, 'Incidence of stuttering among twins,' in W. Johnson and R.R. Leutenegger, eds., *Stuttering in Children and Adults* (Minneapolis, Minn.: University of Minnesota Press 1955)

7 S.E. Nelson, N. Hunter, and M. Walter, 'Stuttering in twin types,' *Journal of Speech Disorders* 10 (1945): 335–43

8 Bloodstein, *Handbook on Stuttering*, 3rd ed., 99

9 L.F. Buscaglia, 'An experimental study of the Sarbin-Hardyck test as indexes of role perception for adolescent stutterers,' *Speech Monographs* 30 (1963): 243

10 C. Cherry and B.McA. Sayers, 'Experiments upon the total inhibition of stammering by external control and some clinical results,' *Journal of Psychosomatic Research* 1 (1956): 233–46

11 C. Van Riper, *Speech Correction: Principles and Methods*, 5th ed. (Englewood Cliffs, NJ: Prentice-Hall 1972), 284

12 J.G. Sheehan and M.M. Martyn, 'Spontaneous recovery from stuttering,' *Journal of Speech and Hearing Research* 9 (1966): 121–35
13 P.J. Glasner and D. Rosenthal, 'Parental diagnosis of stuttering in young children,' *JSHD* 22 (1957): 288–95
14 Sheehan and Martyn, 'Spontaneous recovery from stuttering'; and O. Bloodstein, *A Handbook on Stuttering*, 1st ed. (Chicago, Ill.: National Easter Seals Society 1969), 78–80
15 P.B. Ballard, 'Sinistrality and speech,' *Journal of Experimental Pediatry* 1 (1912): 298–310
16 J.E.W. Wallin, 'A consensus of speech defectives among 89,057 public school pupils – a preliminary report,' *Sch. Soc.* 3 (1916): 213–16
17 Bloodstein, *Handbook on Stuttering*, 3rd ed., 143
18 Ibid., 11
19 Ibid., 18
20 The Hector Speech Aid is manufactured and distributed by Peter Graham Partnership, 10 Eastway, Epsom, Surrey, England KT19 8SG. The author has never used this speech-rate meter and cannot comment on its value.

CHAPTER 3

1 Some speech pathologists and teachers may feel that the classroom trauma described in this chapter is exaggerated. It is true that schools have changed for the better in their treatment of the handicapped. It has also been said that British children are, on the whole, less kind to each other than their North American counterparts. Nevertheless, I still hear about young people with stutters in North America who find their schooling a time of fear, frustration, and humiliation, even in the community colleges where the students are old enough to know better.
2 A.K. Bullen, 'A cross-cultural approach to the problem of stuttering,' *Child Development* 16 (1945): 1–18; and Bloodstein, *Handbook on Stuttering*, 3rd ed., 102
3 J.C. Snidecor, 'Why the Indian does not stutter,' *Quarterly Journal of Speech* 33 (1947): 493–5
4 Ibid.
5 E.M. Lemert, 'Some Indians who stutter,' *JSHD* 18 (1953): 168–74
6 J.L. Stewart, 'The problem of stuttering in certain North American Indian societies,' *JSHD*, Supplement 6 (1960)
7 W. Johnson, *Speech Handicapped School Children* (Minneapolis, Minn.: University of Minnesota Press 1967); and Bloodstein, *Handbook on Stuttering*, 3rd ed., 106–8
8 M.L. Aron, 'The nature and incidence of stuttering among a Bantu group of school-going children,' *JSHD* 27 (1962): 116–28
9 Toyoda, cited in C. Van Riper, *The Nature and Treatment of Stuttering* (Englewood Cliffs, NJ: Prentice-Hall 1971), 39
10 Personal communication, Tokyo Speech Clinic, 1984
11 Bloodstein, *Handbook on Stuttering*, 3rd ed., 80

CHAPTER 4

1 Van Riper, *Speech Correction*, 277
2 H.E. Beech and F. Fransella, *Research and Experiment in Stuttering* (London: Pergamon Press 1968), 55
3 Bloodstein, *Handbook on Stuttering*, 3rd ed., 41–2
4 Ibid., 94
5 Johnson and associates, *The Onset of Stuttering*
6 J. Shields, L.L. Heston, and I.I. Gottesman, 'Schizophrenia and the schizoid: the problem of genetic analysis,' in R.R. Fieve, D. Rosenthal, and H. Brill, eds., *Genetic Research in Psychology* (Baltimore, Md.: Johns Hopkins University Press 1975)
7 S.S. Kety, D. Rosenthal, P.H. Wender, and F. Schulsinger, 'The types and prevalence of mental illness in the biological and adoptive families of adopted schizophrenics,' in D. Rosenthal and S.S. Kety, eds., *The Transmission of Schizophrenia* (Oxford: Pergamon Press 1968), 345–62
8 Bloodstein, *Handbook on Stuttering*, 3rd ed., 98–9
9 Ibid., 101–2
10 L. Chan and B.M. O'Malley, 'Mechanism of action of the sex steroid hormones,' *New England Journal of Medicine* 294 (1976): 1322–8, 1372–81, 1430–7
11 J.P. Scott and J.L. Fuller, *Genetics and the Social Behavior of the Dog* (Chicago, Ill.: University of Chicago Press 1965) Some scientists feel that no form of behaviour is heritable, in spite of mounting evidence to the contrary. Some accept that a nervous disposition may be inherited, but question that specific anxieties (e.g., about speaking) are encoded in our genes. Nevertheless, it is known that young rodents inherit an instinctive fear of a moving shadow overhead (it could be a predatory bird). Even human beings seem to have inherited, from their tree-dwelling ancestors, a fear of falling. This complex subject is discussed in some detail by Melvin Konner, *The Tangled Wing: Biological Constraints on the Human Spirit* (New York: Holt, Rinehart and Winston 1982), 208–35.
12 D.B. Lindsley, 'Bilateral differences in brain potentials from two cerebral hemispheres in relation to laterality and stuttering,' *Journal of Experimental Psychology* 26 (1940): 211–25; and L.C. Douglass, 'The study of laterally recorded EEG's of adult stutterers,' *Journal of Experimental Psychology* 32 (1943): 247–65
13 E. Boberg, L.T. Yeudell, D. Schopflocher, and P. Bo-Lassen, 'The effect of intensive behavioural program on the distribution of EEG alpha power in stutterers during the processing of verbal and visuo-spatial information,' *Journal of Fluency Disorders* 8 (1983): 245–63
14 P.T. Quinn, 'Stuttering, cerebral dominance and the dichotic word test,' *Medical Journal of Australia* 2 (1972): 639–43
15 W.H. Moore and W.O. Haynes, 'Alpha hemispheric asymmetry and stuttering: some support for segmentation dysfunction hypothesis,' *Journal of Speech and Hearing Research* 23 (1980): 229–47

16 Boberg et al., 'Effect of intensive behavioural program on EEG'
17 Bloodstein, *Handbook on Stuttering*, 3rd ed., 10–17
18 R. West, 'An agnostic's speculations about stuttering,' in J. Eisenson, ed., *Stuttering: A Symposium* (New York: Harper and Row 1958)
19 Eisenson, *Stuttering: A Symposium*; and Bloodstein, *Handbook on Stuttering*, 1st ed., 39
20 Konner, *The Tangled Wing*
21 J. Langone, 'Deciphering Dyslexia,' *Discover* (August 1983): 34–42
22 Cherry and Sayers, 'Experiments upon the total inhibition of stammering'; and S. Sutton and R.A. Chase, 'White noise and stuttering,' *Journal of Speech and Hearing Research* 4 (1961): 72
23 C.P. Stromsta, 'A methodology related to the determination of phase angle of bone conducted speech sound energy of stutterers and non-stutterers' (PH D diss., Ohio State University 1956); abstracted in *Speech Monographs* 24 (1957): 147–8
24 Bloodstein, *Handbook on Stuttering*, 3rd ed., 68
25 Ibid., 283–4
26 Ibid., 279
27 G. Fairbanks, 'Systematic research in experimental phonetics I. A theory of the speech mechanism as a servosystem,' *JSHD* 19 (1954): 133–9; and Bloodstein, *Handbook on Stuttering*, 3rd ed., 66–8
28 Bloodstein, *Handbook on Stuttering*, 1st ed., 66–8
29 L.E. Travis and L.B. Fagan, 'Studies in stuttering III. A study of certain reflexes during stuttering,' *Archives of Neurology and Psychiatry* 19 (1928): 1006–13
30 M. Palmer and A.M. Gillett, 'Sex differences in the cardiac rhythms of stutterers,' *Journal of Speech Disorders* 3 (1938): 3–12
31 C.H. Ritzman, 'A comparative cardiovascular and metabolic study of stutterers and non-stutterers,' *Journal of Speech Disorders* 7 (1943): 367–73
32 C.W. Starkweather, 'Stuttering and laryngial behavior – a review,' *ASHA Monographs* (Rockville, Md.: American Speech-Language-Hearing Association, Publication 21, 1982)
33 Beech and Fransella, *Research and Experiment in Stuttering*, 105; and Bloodstein, *Handbook on Stuttering*, 1st ed., 105–6
34 Bloodstein, *Handbook on Stuttering*, 3rd ed., 116–7
35 Beech and Fransella, *Research and Experiment in Stuttering*, 88
36 Ibid.
37 R. Cabanas, 'Some findings in speech and voice therapy among mentally deficient children,' *Folia Phoniat.* 6 (1954): 34–9
38 J.R. Knott, W. Johnson, and M.J. Webster, 'Studies on the psychology of stuttering II. A quantitative evaluation of the expectation of stuttering in relation to the incidence of stuttering,' *Journal of Speech Disorders* 2 (1937): 20–2; and W. Johnson and J.R. Knott, 'The moment of stuttering,' *Journal of Genetic Psychology* 48 (1936): 475–9
39 Bloodstein, *Handbook on Stuttering*, 3rd ed., 44

40 Johnson, *Speech Handicapped School Children*; W. Johnson, 'The role of evaluation in stuttering behavior,' *Journal of Speech Disorders* 3 (1938): 85–9; and Bloodstein, *Handbook on Stuttering*, 3rd ed., 54–6

41 J.G. Sheehan, *Stuttering: Research and Therapy* (New York: Harper and Row 1970)

42 C. Van Riper, *Speech Correction: Principles and Methods*, 3rd ed. (Englewood Cliffs, NJ: Prentice-Hall 1972), 329–30

43 Bloodstein, *Handbook on Stuttering*, 1st ed., 40–5

44 C. Van Riper, 'Study of the thoracic breathing of stutterers during expectancy and occurrence of stuttering spasm,' *Journal of Speech Disorders* 1 (1936): 61–72; Knott, Johnson, and Webster, 'Studies on the psychology of stuttering II'; and R. Milisen, 'Frequency of stuttering with anticipation of stuttering controlled,' *JSHD* 3 (1938): 207–14

45 Bloodstein, *Handbook on Stuttering*, 3rd ed., 224–5

46 E.J. Brutten and B.B. Gray, 'Effect of word cue removal on adaptation and adjacency: a clinical paradigm,'' *JSHD* 26 (1961): 385–9.

47 W. Johnson, R.P. Larson, and J.R. Knott, 'Studies in the psychology of stuttering III. Certain objective cues related to the precipitation of the moment of stuttering,' *JSHD* 2 (1937): 23–5; and A.E. Goss, 'Stuttering behavior and anxiety as a function of experimental training,' *JSHD* 21 (1956): 342–51

48 S.F. Brown, 'The loci of stuttering in the speech sequence,' *Journal of Speech Disorders* 10 (1945): 181–92

49 Bloodstein, *Handbook on Stuttering*, 1st ed., 186

50 S.F. Brown and A. Moren, 'The frequency of stuttering in reading,' *Journal of Speech Disorders* 7 (1942): 153–9

51 Bloodstein, *Handbook on Stuttering*, 1st ed., 193–210

52 N.H. Berwick, 'Stuttering in response to photographs of selected listeners,' in Johnson and Leutenegger, eds., *Stuttering in Children and Adults*

53 J.G. Sheehan, R. Hadley, and E. Gould, 'Impact of authority on stuttering,' *Journal of Abnormal Psychology* 72 (1967): 290–3

54 Bloodstein, *Handbook on Stuttering*, 1st ed., 158

55 H.J. Heltman, *First Aids for Stutterers* (New York: Expression Company 1943)

56 A.E. Goss, 'Stuttering behavior and anxiety as a function of the duration of the stimulus words,' *Journal of Abnormal Social Psychology* 47 (1952): 38–50

57 R.L. Webster, 'A behavioral analysis of stuttering: treatment and theory,' in K. Calhoun, ed., *Innovative Treatment Methods in Psychopathology* (New York: John Wiley and Sons 1974)

CHAPTER 5

1 R.W. Rieber, ed., *The Problem of Stuttering: Theory and Therapy* (New York: Elsevier 1977), 135–6

2 Ibid., 128
3 H. Mercurialis, 'Treatises on the diseases of children,' J. Wollock, trans., in Rieber, ed., *The Problem of Stuttering*, 127–40
4 Ibid.
5 R. Luchsinger and G.E. Arnold, 'Voice speech and language,' in *Clinical Communicology: Its Physiology and Pathology*, 1st ed., G.E. Arnold and E.R. Finkbeiner, trans. (Belmont, Ca.: Wadsworth Publishing 1965), 739–69
6 Ibid.
7 M. Katz, 'Survey of patented anti-stuttering devices,' in Rieber, ed., *The Problem of Stuttering*, 181–206
8 Ibid.
9 Van Riper, *Speech Correction*, 5th ed., 278
10 Ibid., 280
11 H. Geniesse, 'Stuttering,' *Science* 82 (1935): 518
12 Bloodstein, *Handbook on Stuttering*, 3rd ed., 250
13 Beech and Fransella, *Research and Experiment in Stuttering*, 171
14 V. Meyer and J.M. Mair, 'A new technique to control stammering: a preliminary report,' *Behaviour Research and Therapy* 1 (1963): 251–4
15 Ibid.; and Beech and Fransella, *Research and Experiment in Stuttering*, 176
16 I. Goldiamond, 'Stuttering and fluency as manipulatable operant response classes,' in L. Krasner and L.P. Ulman, eds., *Research in Behavior Modification* (New York: Holt, Rinehart and Winston 1965); and G.A. Soderburg, 'Delayed auditory feedback and stuttering,' *JSHD* 33 (1968): 260–7
17 A. Dewar, A.D. Dewar, and H.E. Barnes, 'Automatic triggering of auditory feedback masking in stammering and cluttering,' *British Journal of Disorders of Communication* 11 (1976): 19–26
18 A. Dewar, A.D. Dewar, W.T.S. Austin, and H.M. Brash, 'The long-term use of an automatically triggered auditory feedback device in the treatment of stammering,' *British Journal of Disorders of Communication* 14: 3 (1978): 219–29
19 Ibid.
20 Ibid.
21 J.G. Sheehan, 'Reflections on the behavioral modification of stuttering,' in M. Fraser, ed., *Conditioning in Stuttering Therapy – Applications and Limitations* (Memphis, Tenn.: Speech Foundation of America, Publication 7, 1981), 123–36
22 Beech and Fransella, *Research and Experiment in Stuttering*, 91–6
23 United States Pharmacopeial Convention, Inc., *About Your Medicines* (Kingsport Press: distributed in Canada by Canadian Pharmaceutical Association 1981), 336–9, 235–8, 297–301; and J. Graedon, *The People's Pharmacy* (New York: St Martin's Press 1976), 47, 269
24 Van Riper, *Speech Correction*, 5th ed., 333–5
25 A.A. Brill, 'Speech disturbances in nervous and mental disease,' *Quarterly Journal of Speech Education* 9 (1923): 129–35

226 Notes to pages 103-16

26 Beech and Fransella, *Research and Experiment in Stuttering*, 105-24
27 C. Tavris, *Anger: The Misunderstood Emotion* (New York: Simon and Schuster 1982), 121-50
28 Van Riper, *Speech Correction*, 5th ed., 275
29 Bloodstein, *Handbook on Stuttering*, 1st ed., 241-2
30 J. Hoffman, 'The application of Gestalt therapy principles to therapy with an adult stutterer' (Mimeo abstract, Ontario Speech and Hearing Convention 1976)
31 J.B. Watson, *Behaviorism* (New York: W.W. Norton 1924, cited in Konner, *The Tangled Wing*, 219
32 Konner, *The Tangled Wing*, 383-4
33 B. Flanagan, I. Goldiamond, and N. Azrin, 'Operant stuttering: the control of stuttering behavior through response-contingent consequences,' *Journal of Experimental Analysis of Behavior* 1 (1958): 173-7
34 R.R. Martin and G.M. Siegel, 'The effects of response contingent shock on stuttering,' *Journal of Speech and Hearing Research* 9 (1966): 340-52; and 'The effects of simultaneously punishing stuttering and rewarding fluency, *Journal of Speech and Hearing Research* 9 (1966): 466-75; and B. Biggs and J. Sheehan, 'Punishment or distraction? Operant stuttering revisited,' *Journal of Abnormal Psychology* (1970), cited in Bloodstein, *Handbook on Stuttering*, 3rd ed., 50
35 Fraser, ed., *Conditioning in Stuttering Therapy*, 12, 132
36 B. Guitar and T. Peters, *Stuttering: An Integration of Contemporary Therapies* (Memphis, Tenn.: Speech Foundation of America, Publication 16, 1980), 13
37 Webster, 'A behavioral analysis of stuttering'; also R.L. Webster, 'Empirical considerations regarding stuttering therapy,' in H.H. Gregory, ed., *Controversies about Stuttering Therapy* (Baltimore, Md.: University Park Press 1979)
38 Bloodstein, *Handbook on Stuttering*, 3rd ed., 365-6
39 B.P. Ryan, *Programmed Therapy for Stuttering in Young Children* (Springfield, Ill.: Charles C. Thomas 1974); 'Stuttering therapy in a framework of operant conditioning and programmed learning,' in Gregory, ed., *Controversies about Stuttering Therapy*, 129-73; Webster, 'A behavioral analysis of stuttering'; and Webster, 'Empirical considerations regarding stuttering therapy'
40 F.L. Darley and D.C. Spriestersbach, *Diagnostic Methods in Speech Pathology* (New York: Harper and Row 1978)
41 Guitar and Peters, *Stuttering*, 33-6
42 Bloodstein, *Handbook on Stuttering*, 3rd ed., 343-53
43 W. Johnson, *People in Quandaries* (New York: Harper and Row 1946); Johnson, 'The time, the place and the problem,' in Johnson and Leutenegger, eds., *Stuttering in Children and Adults*; and Bloodstein, *Handbook on Stuttering*, 3rd ed., 347-9
44 C. Van Riper, 'Experiments in stuttering therapy,' in Eisenson, ed., *Stuttering: A Symposium*

45 Van Riper, *Speech Correction*, 5th ed., 248–340
46 Ibid., 291–2
47 Ibid., 292
48 E. Boberg and D. Kully, *Clinical Manual for Comprehensive Stutter-ing Program* (Edmonton, Alberta: University of Alberta 1984); and E. Boberg, 'Intensive adult therapy program,' *Seminars in Speech, Language and Hearing* 1: 4 (1980): 365–73
49 E. Boberg, ed., *The Maintenance of Fluency*. Proceedings of the Banff Conference, Banff, Alberta, June 1979 (New York: Elsevier 1981); and Boberg, *Clinical Manual*
50 G. Andrews, B. Guitar, and P. Howie, 'Meta-analysis of the effects of stuttering treatment,' *JSHD* 45 (1980): 287–307

CHAPTER 6

1 ASHA is essentially a professional association, but has a consumer branch called the National Association for Hearing and Speech Action (NAHSA) at 10801 Rockville Pike, Rockville, Maryland 20852, U.S.A. Telephone: (301) 638-6868 and (301) 897-8682. Helpline: (800) 638-8255 (or 6868). This is an active organization with a full-time staff.
2 The Canadian Speech and Hearing Association (CSHA) is a profes-sional organization, but the local branches will point stutterers toward suitable clinics. There is a need for a consumer-oriented branch in Canada.
3 M. Fraser, ed., *To the Stutterer* (Memphis, Tenn.: Speech Founda-tion of America, Publication 9, 1972); and *Self-Therapy for the Stut-terer*, 3rd ed. (Memphis, Tenn.: Speech Foundation of America, Publication 12, 1981); Malcolm Fraser has written and edited many excellent publications for the Speech Foundation of America in Memphis, Tennessee. Many of these are designed for use by non-professionals.
4 S. Ainsworth, *Counselling Stutterers* (Memphis, Tenn.: Speech Foun-dation of America n.d.)
5 A. Irwin, *Stammering: Practical Help for All Ages* (Markham, Ont.: Penguin Books 1980)
6 National Stuttering Project, 1269 7th Avenue, San Francisco, California 94122. Telephone: (415) 566-5324 or (415) 647-4700. Issues a newsletter.
7 R.L. Gregory, 'Recovery from early blindness: a case study,' in R.L. Gregory, ed., *Concepts and Mechanisms of Perception* (London: Duckworth 1974), 65–129
8 R.M. Restak, *The Brain: The Last Frontier* (New York: Warner Books 1979), 96–102, 407–9. Excerpts by permission of Doubleday & Co., Inc. Copyright 1979, Richard M. Restak.

CHAPTER 7

1 Webster, 'A behavioral analysis of stuttering'

CHAPTER 8

1 The inevitability of sibling rivalry in the family was questioned by one reviewer. She pointed out that my childhood was spent in Britain and that British children tend to be more unkind to each other than North American children. This may be true, but from what I know of human nature and with experience of how small brothers and sisters compete and call each other names, I feel that the rivalries are usually there. It is just a matter of degree.
2 Bloodstein, *Handbook on Stuttering*, 3rd ed., 108–9
3 L.J. Peter, *Peter's Quotations: Ideas for Our Time* (Toronto, London, New York: Bantam Books 1979), 57

CHAPTER 9

1 J. Levy, 'Perception of bilateral chimeric figures following hemispheric disconnection,' *Brain* 95 (1972): 61–78; 'The origins of lateral symmetry,' in *Lateralization in the Nervous System* (New York: Academic Press 1977); and Interview with J. Levy described in J. Restak, *The Brain*
2 F.H.C. Crick, 'Thinking about the brain,' *Scientific American* 241: 3 (1979): 219–32
3 C.F. Stevens, 'The neuron,' *Scientific American* 241: 3 (1979): 54–65
4 N. Geschwind, 'Specializations of the human brain,' *Scientific American* 241: 3 (1979): 180–99
5 J.P. Mohr, cited in Geschwind, 'Specializations of the human brain'
6 Geschwind, 'Specializations of the human brain'
7 J.A. Gray, *The Psychology of Fear and Stress* (New York: McGraw-Hill 1971); and Konner, *The Tangled Wing*, 220–1
8 Konner, *The Tangled Wing*, 220–5
9 Ibid., 223–7
10 J.F. Tallman, S.M. Paul, P. Skolnick, and D.W. Gallagher, 'Receptors for the age of anxiety: pharmacology of the Benzodiapines,' *Science* 207 (1980): 274–81
11 Webster, 'A behavioral analysis of stuttering'
12 W.M. Shearer, 'Speech: behavior of middle-ear muscle during stuttering,' *Science* 152 (1966): 1280; and Webster, 'A behavioral analysis of stuttering'
13 Webster, 'A behavioral analysis of stuttering'
14 B.B. Brown, *Stress and the Art of Biofeedback* (Toronto: Bantam Books 1981), 65–6
15 B. Guitar, 'Reduction of stuttering frequency using analog electromyographic feedback,' *Journal of Speech and Hearing Research* 18 (1975): 672–85
16 Bloodstein, *Handbook on Stuttering*, 3rd. ed., 366–7
17 M. Karlins and L.M. Andrews, *Biofeedback: Turning on the Power of Your Mind* (New York: Warner Books 1976), 57

Glossary

Anyone who attempts to define the terms used in psychology, neurology, pharmacology, and speech therapy is sure to get into hot water, but it is essential that a reader knows precisely what the author means when he uses unfamiliar words. Many glossaries, dictionaries, and textbooks were consulted to try to tie down precise meanings of words, but few experts seemed to say the same thing.

The words in this glossary are defined in the sense that they are used in this book and some are explained in more detail in the text. There are other meanings, and shades of meaning, and some definitions are over-simplified or over-generalized. The word 'stuttering,' for example, has three pages of definitions in Malcolm Fraser's glossary (see the following paragraph), and the psychologists seem to have difficulty saying exactly what the words 'psychologist,' 'psychiatrist,' and 'psychotherapy' mean.

Readers interested in a wider vocabulary about stuttering are referred to Malcolm Fraser's excellent booklet, *Stuttering Words – A Glossary of the Meanings of Words and Terms Used or Associated with Stuttering and Speech Pathology* (Memphis, Tenn.: Speech Foundation of America, Publication 2, 1980).

albumins A group of proteins soluble in water and coagulated by heat.

ambidextrous, ambidextrality The ability to use either hand with equal efficiency.

anticipatory struggle The abnormal feelings and behaviour of a stutterer as he prepares to speak and tries to avoid expected speech difficulties.

aphasia Partial or complete loss of the ability to speak in a comprehensive way, to understand spoken words, and to formulate, understand or express meanings as a result of injury, disease, or other abnormalities of the brain.

auditory feedback The sensations produced by the stimulation of the ear by the sound of one's own speech transmitted by air or bone.

axon The nerve fibre that transmits messages from one nerve cell (neuron) to another. The axon transmits; the dendrites receive (see 'dendrites' and 'neuron').

Broca's area (or **Broca's convolution**) The area in the brain responsible for programming the speech signals to the brain's motor tissues that control the movements of lips, tongue, jaw, larynx, etc. Sometimes called the speech area.

cerebral dominance The dominance of one side of the brain's cerebral cortex for a particular function (e.g., speech). See also 'laterality.'

chlorpromazine A phenothiazine drug used to treat nervous, mental, and emotional disorders.

cluttering Rapid, jerky, disjointed speech, with slurred or jumbled articulation. Thought to be due to a neurological disorder.

cognitive mismatch A mismatch between what a child sees or hears on one occasion and what he has experienced before.

conditioning Procedures used to elicit specific responses to situations, objects, etc., in order to modify behaviour. In general it means 'learning.'

creatinine A chemical compound (methylglycocyamidine) in muscle and urine.

creative dramatics Use of drama in psychotherapy and speech therapy to identify areas of conflict and provide release by playing roles.

decibel (Db) A unit of sound-wave intensity.

delayed auditory feedback The hearing of one's speech after a brief time interval.

dendrites Fine branches of the nerve cell (neuron) that receive signals from other nerves.

desensitization See 'systematic desensitization.'

disfluency Speech that is not smooth and fluent to a degree that can be normal (all people hesitate when they speak) or excessive (as in a stutter).

distraction Diverting the attention from the speech and thereby reducing the speaker's fear of stuttering.

dyslexia A perceptual disorder making it difficult for a person to read, write, spell, and, in some cases, speak.

easy onset Starting a sound, syllable, or word slowly and gradually without tension. Synonymous with 'easy initiation.'

echo speech See 'shadowing.'

Edinburgh Masker A portable electronic instrument that prevents a stutterer from hearing himself as he speaks.

endocrine glands Glands that secrete and release hormones (e.g., adrenalin and insulin) that affect the organs of the body.

epilepsy A disorder of the nervous system involving periodic fits, paroxysms, and loss of consciousness.

etiology The predisposition, development, and maintenance of a complaint (e.g., a stutter).

extrovert A person with an attitude that directs the consciousness towards the external objective world (antonym = 'introvert'). Jung recognized a distinct, extroverted type.

eye contact Looking the listener in the eye while speaking to him, and receiving visual feedback.

fluency shaping therapy Speech therapy that applies benign conditioning techniques to modify the speech behaviour of stutterers (easy onset to words, prolongation of sounds) by graded tasks, without treating the origins of the stutter or the anxiety about speaking.

fricative Sound made by forcing air through an orifice narrowed by tongue and lip movement (e.g., 'th,' 'f,' 'v,' and the sibilants 's,' 'z,' 'sh').

general semantics The relationships between the language people use and the way they act. Used in speech therapy to define and treat a stutterer's false assumptions about his speech.

Gestalt psychology A system of psychology concerned with patterns and the whole person.

globulins A group of proteins that dissolve in salt solutions but not in water (globulin, fibrinogens, fibrin, etc).

hertz (Hz) A unit of frequency of one cycle per second.

incus (anvil) A bone shaped like a tooth with two roots. Located in the middle ear.

introvert A person with an attitude that directs the consciousness toward the inner, subjective world. (Antonym = 'extrovert'). Jung recognized a distinct introverted type.

laterality The relationship between brain-sidedness and left- and right-handedness and speech. The 'laterality theory' is that a shift in handedness or confusion in sidedness is involved in the onset and maintenance of stuttering. See 'cerebral dominance.'

learned behaviour A persistent change in the responses of nerves, muscles, emotions, speech, and behaviour in response to external stimuli in the environment and clinic.

malleus (hammer) A small bone with an oval head and spur located in the middle ear.

masker An instrument emitting a sound used in masking to prevent the speaker hearing his own speech (e.g., 'Edinburgh Masker').

masking Interference with the perception of sound by the ears so that the speaker cannot hear his own speech. Sometimes used in the sense of changing the patterns and quality of sound the speaker hears.

masseter An elevator muscle of the lower jaw.

meprobamate A systemic drug used to treat nervousness and tension.

middle ear (tympanum) The part of the ear just inside the ear-drum that contains the three-boned lever (ossicular chain), and the muscles that control and support it, involved in the amplification and transmission of sound to the inner-ear membrane.

motor cortex The parts of the brain concerned with movement of lips, tongue, head, limbs, etc.

mute A person who cannot speak.

myelin A white fatty substance that forms the protective sheath of nerve fibres (axons).

neuroleptic drug A drug that affects the central nervous system's chemicals ('neurotransmitters') that transmit messages across the junction of one nerve with another.

neuron A nerve cell. Neurons are the building blocks of the brain. Each one consists of a roughly spherical or pyramidal cell body with numerous fine branches (dendrites) radiating from it and receiving signals from other nerve cells. A nerve fibre (the axon) extends from the cell body and transmits signals to other nerves.

neurosis A personality disorder causing a person to have irrational fears, obsessions, and compulsions, and preventing him from dealing effectively with reality.

neurotransmitters The chemical compounds that carry the nerve signals across the synaptic gap where one nerve cell connects with another (e.g., dopamine).

nonfluency See 'disfluency.'

non-verbal communication Messages conveyed not by spoken or written words but by involuntary movements of the face and limbs and by posture.

operant conditioning The form of conditioning in which a person's response allows reinforcement of behaviour (i.e., rewarded behaviour is likely to be positively reinforced and punished behaviour negatively reinforced).

ossicular chain The chain of small bones (the malleus, incus, and stapes) involved in sound transmission and amplification in the middle ear.

perseveration The abnormal persistence of a mental or motor (movement) process after the situation that caused it has ceased to exist.

phenobarbitone (or **phenobarbital**) A drug that depresses the activity of the central nervous system.

phobia An excessive, irrational anxiety about an object or situation.

phonetics The science of speech sounds.

play therapy The use of play activities in the psychotherapy and speech therapy of children.

plosive A sound created by interrupting air flow, building up air pressure, and releasing it, as in 'd,' 'b,' 'p,' 't,' etc.

preparatory set The hidden and often involuntary preparation or rehearsal for speech by pre-setting the positions of lips, tongue, etc.

prolongation The lengthening of speech sounds or lip, tongue, etc., postures.

propositional speech Speech containing meaning and implication.

psychiatrist An expert who applies specialized knowledge to treat mental and nervous disorders; covers both psychotherapy and psychology. *Note*: In this book the word refers to practitioners with a medical degree (MD).

psychobiology The study of psychology in terms of biological brain processes.

psychologist An expert who applies psychology for therapeutic purposes. *Note*: In this book the word refers to practitioners without a medical qualification (MD).

psychotherapy Treatment of mental illness, personality maladjustments, and harmful attitudes by psychological means.

pull-out Voluntary, controlled release from a stuttering block.

rhythmic therapy Treatment of stuttering using rhythm (a metronome, marching, etc.) as part of the speaking pattern. Regarded by many as a form of distraction.

schizophrenia A mental disorder involving conflicts between or separation of different aspects of personality and affecting the emotions and behaviour.

semantics The scientific study of the meaning of words.

shadowing Speaking at the same time as another person, or with a slight delay. Synonymous with 'echo speech.'

sociobiology The biology of social behaviour.

stammering See 'stuttering.'

stapedius A small muscle in the middle ear.

stapes (the stirrup) A stirrup-shaped small bone in the middle ear.

stematil One of the phenothiazine drugs used to control nervous, emotional, and mental conditions.

stuttering A speech disorder consisting of excessive and conspicuous involuntary hesitations, repetitions, prolongations, and blocks that interrupt the speech flow, together with struggling to speak, anxiety about speaking, and avoidance of words and speaking situations. *Note*: There are many other definitions.

stuttering modification therapy Speech therapy designed to reduce avoidance of speaking and hard words, lessen anxieties about speech, modify attitudes about speech, and help the stutterer change his pattern of disfluency.

synapse The connection of one nerve cell to another. At the junction there is a gap across which chemical compounds (neurotransmitters) carry the nerve signal.

syndrome A group of symptoms typical of a complaint (e.g., a stutter).

systematic desensitization Weakening of an undesirable response by repeated, gradual exposure to the situations that cause it.

tensor tympani A small muscle in the middle ear.

tympanum See 'middle ear.'

voluntary controlled repetition (VCR) The deliberate, voluntary, repetition of a sound, syllable, or word in a smooth, prolonged effortless manner to replace uncontrolled, involuntary repetition (stuttering) and reduce fear and avoidance of speaking.

voluntary stuttering See 'voluntary controlled repetition (VCR).'

Wernicke's area The tissue in the brain responsible for language formulation and comprehension.

Suggested reading

The Speech Foundation of America Publications described below can be purchased for about $1.50 to $2.00 (U.S.) from the Director, Speech Foundation of America, 152 Lombardy Rd., Memphis, Tennessee 38111.

General Reviews

Bloodstein, Oliver. *A Handbook on Stuttering.* 3rd edition. Chicago, Ill.: National Easter Seals Society for Crippled Children and Adults 1981
   This is a first-class review. The approach is technical, but the book is written in simple English and is easy to understand.
Van Riper, Charles. *The Nature of Stuttering.* Englewood Cliffs, NJ: Prentice-Hall, Inc. 1971
   A very readable general treatment of stuttering.
– *Speech Correction: Principles and Methods.* 5th edition. Englewood Cliffs, NJ: Prentice-Hall, Inc. 1972.
   Describes many speech defects and their treatment. Aimed at clinicians, but the simple style will appeal to the layman.

Guidance for Parents with Stuttering Children

Ainsworth, Stanley. *Stuttering: What It Is and What to Do about It.* Lincoln, Neb.: Cliff's Notes n.d.
   A low-cost booklet giving more details than the following publication.
Ainsworth, Stanley and J. Fraser-Gruss. *If Your Child Stutters – A Guide for Parents.* Revised edition. Memphis, Tenn.: Speech Foundation of America, Publication 11, 1977

An excellent low-cost summary written for the layman.
Available from the Speech Foundation of America, Memphis,
Tenn.

Self-help

Barbara, Dominick A. *A Practical Self-Help Guide for
Stutterers*. Springfield, Ill.: Charles C. Thomas 1983.
Useful counsel about attitudes.
Fraser, Malcolm. *Self-therapy for the Stutterer*. Revised edition.
Memphis, Tenn.: Speech Foundation of America, Publication
12, 1981.
Probably the best book on self-help. Its cost is low, it is
simply written, and up to date. See also several articles in:
Fraser, Malcolm, ed. *To the Stutterer*. Memphis, Tenn.:
Speech Foundation of America, Publication 9, 1972.

Guidance for Teachers and School Clinicians

Fraser, Malcolm, *Stuttering – Treatment of the Young in School*.
Memphis, Tenn.: Speech Foundation of America, Publication
4, 1982.
Mainly written for public-school speech therapists, it pro-
vides the non-specialist with guidance about what to do and
what not to do when dealing with stuttering children.
Leith, William R. *Handbook of Stuttering – Therapy for the
School Clinician*. San Diego, Ca.: College Hill Press 1980

Guidance for Stutterers

Fraser, Malcolm, ed. *To the Stutterer*. Memphis, Tenn.: Speech
Foundation of America, Publication 9, 1972
A remarkable, encouraging book written by twenty-five
experts. Covers attitudes, therapy, self-help, and dealing with
fear.

Modern Views and Therapies

Curlee, Richard F. and William H. Perkins, eds.
Nature and Treatment of Stuttering. New Directions. San
Diego, Ca.: College Hill Press 1984

An up-to-date review of the treatment of stuttering.
Describes promising methods for the future. Valuable for the
clinician and informed layman.

Ingham, Roger J. *Stuttering and Behaviour Therapy – Current
Status and Experimental Foundations.* San Diego, Ca.: College
Hill Press 1983

A first-class review of treatment for stuttering written
mainly for the clinician but also useful for the informed
layman.

Self-help and consumer organizations

Self-help organizations tend to come and go, but there are a few hard-core national organizations that have many local chapters. These organizations create opportunities for timid stutterers to come out into the open and meet people who will not mock their strange way of speaking. They provide a forum for airing feelings, views, and complaints, and opportunities to test newly learned ways of speaking. These groups help to dispel the loneliness of many stutterers trapped in their glass towers.

A stutterer who is fearful about approaching a doctor about his problem but who wants to be helped will find that these organizations, some of which have clinicians as members, are a good starting-point. He is likely to be greeted with sympathy and understanding, and will be given gentle but hard-nosed advice.

The addresses given are those provided in 1984. They tend to change.

SELF-HELP ORGANIZATIONS

Australia

Australian Speak Easy
  Association
PO Box 113
Maclean
New South Wales 2463

Speak Easy Association
Victoria Branch
GPO 1173 K
Melbourne, Victoria 3001

Speak Easy Association
New South Wales and
ACT Branch
PO Box 1004
Parramatta
New South Wales 2150
(Speak Easy has branches in
other parts of Australia.)

Canada

Speak Easy, Inc.
95 Evergreen Avenue
Saint John, New Brunswick
E2N 1H4
Telephone: (506) 696-6799
Newsletter: *Speaking Out*
(There are several local
branches)

L'Association des bégues du
Canada (l'ABC)
3600 Fullum 26
Montreal, Québec H2K 3P6
Newsletter: *Speaking Out*

Denmark

P-Klub, Föreningen for
Stammere i Denmark,
(P-Club, Association for
Stutterers in Denmark)
c/o Taleinstitutte
Tjornevej 6
DK-8240, Risskov

Finland

Finska Stammares Förening rf.
(National Association of
Finnish Stutterers)
Box 60
SF-00131, Helsinki

Japan

Japanese Association of
Stutterers for Help and
Friendship
Shinjo Fukano
A-44-306 Khoro 5
Otokoyama, Yahata-shi
Kyoto 614

Norway

Norsk Interesseorganisasjon
for Stamme (NIFS)
(Norwegian Fellow-
Organization for Stutterers)
Postbox 878
Sentrum, N-Oslo 1

Sweden

SSR (Sveriges Stamnings-
föreningars Riksförbund)
(Stutterers' Clubs Organization
of Sweden)
Box 755
S-101 30 Stockholm 1
(There are eleven local chapters
of the Swedish P-Club:
Blekinge, Dalarna, Göteborg,
Norrboten, Jönköping,

Upplands, Kronoberg, Skåne,
Stockholm, Västmanlands,
and Östergötland.)

Switzerland

Vereinigung für Stotternde
und Angehörige (Versta)
Postfach 437
CH 8042, Zurich

United Kingdom

Association for Stammerers
21a Pound Lane
Epsom, Surrey
(Several local chapters.)

Association for Stammerers
86 Blackfriars Road
London SE1 8HA
Newsletter: *Speaking Out*

United States

National Stuttering Project
1269 7th Avenue
San Francisco, California
94122
Telephone: (415) 566-5324 and
647-4700
Newsletter: *Letting Go*
(There are many branches of
this organization in the
United States.)

National Council of Adult
Stutterers
Speech and Hearing Clinic

Catholic University of America
Washington, DC 20064
Telephone: (202) 635-5556

Council for Adult Stutterers
11435 Monterrey Drive
Silver Spring, Maryland 20902

National Association of
Councils of Stutterers
1724 North Troy Street
Nr. 772
Arlington, Virginia 22201

Speakeasy International
233 Concord Drive
Paramus, New Jersey 07652

West Germany

Der Kieselstein (The Pebble)
Mitteilungsblatt Deutsch-
sprachiger Stotterergruppen
Bundesvereinigung Stotterer-
Selbsthilfe
Baustrasse 2
5650 Solingen 11
Newsletter: *Der Kieselstein*
(Chapters in forty-two German
cities.)

Bundesvereinigung Stotterer-
Selbsthilfe
Postfach 110222
5650 Solingen 11
Telephone: 02122-73075

CONSUMER ORGANIZATIONS

There are two consumer-related organizations in the United
States that provide information and advice for stutterers. They
both have full-time staff and provide excellent service.

National Association for Hearing and Speech Action (NAHSA)
10801 Rockville Pike
Rockville, Maryland 20852
Telephone: (301) 638-6868 and 897-8682
Helpline: 800-638-8255 (or 6868)

The seventy-year-old NAHSA is the consumer affiliate of the
professional American Speech-Language-Hearing Association
(ASHA). NAHSA deals with communication disorders in general,
including deafness, aphasia, and stuttering. The Helpline
telephone link provides toll-free communication with the experts.

A small annual fee is charged for members. The group
enables people with communication disorders to influence
government policy, keep informed about the most modern types
of treatment and new devices, tap NAHSA's extensive information
system about speech disorders, and become part of a network of
people working to help people who cannot communicate effectively. A newsletter, *NAHSA News*, is published quarterly.

The Speech Foundation of America
152 Lombardy Road
Memphis, Tennessee 38111
Telephone: (901) 452-0995

The Speech Foundation of America provides advice and publishes low-cost booklets about speech disorders, particularly
stuttering. Some of the booklets are for clinicians, but many are
designed to advise and help parents and teachers of stuttering
children and the stutterers themselves. The booklets are well
written in simple language and contain sound advice.

Parents bewildered by their children's speech behaviour but
reluctant to approach a clinician will find some of the booklets
invaluable.

Both of these organizations provide people who have speech
and hearing defects with a first-class lifeline. It is hoped that
similar organizations will develop in other countries.

Organizations concerned with stuttering therapy and research

The organizations in different countries concerned with stuttering and other speech disorders are listed below to provide points of contact for those interested in treatment and the more technical aspects of speech pathology. Some organizations are professional associations for speech pathologists; and others are involved in research, or treatment, or both.

It would be impossible to list all the centres. There are about 24,000 clinicians treating speech disorders in the United States alone. The centres listed are to some extent chosen arbitrarily and reflect the replies to a one-year survey carried out with the help of the different embassies. No information is provided about the quality of the therapy provided. The larger hospitals treat stuttering in most countries, but the degree of specialization and type of therapy vary considerably.

There are many private clinics and free-lance therapists, but it should be remembered that the objective of most of these private enterprises is to make money. Some of these commercial establishments are genuine and helpful, but a person with a stutter seeking help should get professional advice before spending his money on treatment that may at best provide only a short-term benefit, and may at worst do lasting damage. *Caveat emptor*!

International

General Secretary
International Association of
  Logopedics and Phoniatrics
  (IALP)

European Chairman:
Dr E.F. Stournaras
Erasmus University
Overschiese Kleiweg 498
3045 PS Rotterdam
Netherlands

North American Chairman:
  Dr E. Conture
400 Scott Avenue
Syracuse, New York 13210
U.S.A.

Australia

Australian Association of
  Speech and Hearing
253 Hampton Street
Hampton, Victoria 3188
Telephone: 598-0097

Prince Henry Hospital
Anzac Parade
Little Bay
New South Wales 2036
Telephone: 661-0111

Cumberland College Health
  Sciences
PO Box 170
Lidcombe
New South Wales 2141
Telephone: 646-6444

Office of the Principal
South Australia College of
  Advanced Education
46 Kintore Avenue
Adelaide
South Australia 5000
Telephone: 08-228-1611

Most states in Australia have
several clinics that specialize in
stuttering therapy. The speech
pathology departments of most
major hospitals will direct
people to centres for advice,
information, and treatment.

Austria

Arbeitsgemeinschaft
  Österreichischer Phoniater
p.A. OA Dr med H. Hoffer
II HND-Univers. Klinik
Garnissongasse 13
A 1090 Wien

Österreichische Gesellschaft für
  Logopadie, Phoniatrie, und
  Pädaudiologie
I HND-Univers. Klinik
Dept. Phoniatrie
Lazarettg. 14, A 1090 Wien
Telephone: 4800-3316,
  3317 DW

These are the addresses of the
professional organizations of
speech specialists in Austria.
Stutterers are treated at the
ear, nose, and throat clinics of
the major hospitals, and there
are no special centres for
speech therapy.

Belgium

French-speaking Area
Centre du Langage
Service d'oto-rhino-
  laryngologie
Cliniques Universitaire St
  Pierre
1000 Bruxelles

Service de Rééducation de la
  Parole et du Langage
Service d'oto-rhino-
  laryngologie
l'Hôpital de Bavière
Université de Liège
Bld de la Constitution
4000 Liège

Centre Universitaire d'Audio-
  Phonologie Paul Guns
Clos Chapelle aux Champs 30
BTE 30, 40
1200 Bruxelles
Telephone: 762-34-00
  Ext. 32.40

Flemish-speaking Area
Katholieke Universiteit (Speech
  Pathology)
Leuven

Vrije Universiteit
  (Neurolinguistics)
Brussel

Katholieke Vlaamse Hoge-
  school
J. De Bomstraat 11
2000 Antwerpen

HIPB (Speech Pathology)
St-Lievenspoortstraat 143
9000 Gent

HRIPB (Speech Pathology)
De Pintelaan 135
9000 Gent

HTI (Speech Pathology)
Spoorwegstraat 12
8200 Brugge

Vlaamse Verenining voor
  Logopedisten
Antwerpsesteenweg 154
2350 Vosselaar

Federatie voor Revalidatie-
  centra
Kasteelstraat
2700 Sint-Niklaas

Rehabilitation Centre for
  Speech and Hearing
  Disorders
UZ St-Rafael

Canada

Alberta
Alberta Speech and Hearing
  Association
308 Corbett Hall
University of Alberta
Edmonton T6G 0T2

Department of Speech
  Pathology
411 Garneau Professional
  Building
University of Alberta
Edmonton T6G 0T2

Department of Speech
  Pathology and Audiology
University of Alberta
400-11044 82 Avenue
Edmonton T6G 0T2
Telephone: (403) 432-5990

Department of Neuro-
  psychology
PO Box 307, Alberta Hospital
Edmonton T5J 2J7

Stuttering Clinic
Department of Speech
  Pathology and Audiology
University of Alberta Hospitals
83rd Avenue and 112th Street
Edmonton T6G 2B7

Alberta Society for Stuttering
  Research
c/o Department of Speech
  Pathology
400 Garneau Professional
  Centre
University of Alberta
Edmonton T6G 0T2

Alberta Children's Hospital
1820 Richmond Road SW
Calgary T2T 5C7

British Columbia
British Columbia Speech and
  Hearing Association
2125 West 7th Avenue
Vancouver V6K 1X9

Speech Pathology Department
Lions Gate Hospital
230 East 13th Street
North Vancouver V7L 2L7

South Okanagan Health Unit
PO Box 340, Kelly Avenue
Summerland V0H 1Z0

Manitoba
Manitoba Speech and Hearing
  Association
PO Box 474
Winnipeg R3C 2J3
Telephone: (204) 489-7143

Speech Therapy Department
Seven Oaks General Hospital
2300 McPhillips Street
Winnipeg R2V 3M3

New Brunswick
New Brunswick Speech and
  Hearing Association
180 Woodbridge Street
Fredericton E3B 4R3

Speech Therapy Department
St John Regional Hospital
PO Box 2100
St John E2L 4L2

Newfoundland
Newfoundland Speech and
  Hearing Association
PO Box 8201, Postal Station
  'A'
St John's A1B 3N4

Speech Pathology Department
L.A. Miller Centre
Forest Road
St John's A1A 1E5

Speech Pathology Department
Sir Thomas Roddick Hospital
Stephenville A2N 2V6

Nova Scotia
Speech and Hearing
  Association of Nova Scotia
PO Box 775, Postal Station
  'M'
Halifax B3J 2V2

Speech and Hearing
  Association of Nova Scotia
PO Box 975
Truro B2N 5G8
Telephone: (902) 895-1511

Nova Scotia Hearing and
  Speech Clinic
Fenwick Place
5599 Fenwick Street
Halifax B3H 1R2

Speech Clinic
Yarmouth Regional Hospital
Yarmouth B5A 2P5

Ontario
Canadian Speech and Hearing
  Association
Royal York Hotel
Convention Mezzanine
100 Front Street
Toronto M5J 1E3
Telephone: (416) 368-8132

Disfluency Program
Speech and Language
  Pathology
Children's Hospital of Eastern
  Ontario
401 Smyth Road
PO Box 8010
Ottawa K1H 8L1
Telephone: (613) 737-7600

Communication Disorders
Royal Ottawa Regional
  Rehabilitation Centre
505 Smyth Road
Ottawa K1H 8M2
Telephone: (613) 737-7350

Precision Fluency Shaping
  Program
Clarke Institute
Speech Pathology Department
250 College Street
Toronto M5T 1R8
Telephone: (416) 979-2221

Speech Pathology
Department of Rehabilitation
Toronto General Hospital
101 College Street
Toronto M5G 1L7

Speech Pathology Department
Hospital for Sick Children
555 University Avenue
Toronto M5G 1X8
Telephone: (416) 597-1500

Department of Language
  Pathology
University of Western Ontario
339 Windermere Road
PO Box 5339, Postal Station
  'A'
London N6A 5A5

Speech Pathology
Scarborough General Hospital
3050 Lawrence Avenue East
Scarborough M1P 2V5
Telephone: (416) 438-2911

Many of the school boards and major hospitals in Ontario are concerned with speech disorders.

Prince Edward Island
Prince Edward Island Speech
 and Hearing Association
c/o Department of Health and
 Social Services
Social Services Branch
PO Box 2000
Charlottetown C1A 7N8

Co-ordinator, Speech and
 Hearing Program
Department of Social Services
PO Box 2000
Charlottetown C1A 7N8

Quebec
Le Corporation professionelle
 des orthophonistes et
 audiologistes du Québec
4770 rue de Salaberry
Montreal H4J 1H6
Telephone: (514) 332-9090

School of Human
 Communication Disorders
McGill University
1266 Pine Avenue West
Montreal H3A 1A1

Department of Speech
 Pathology and Audiology
Montreal General Hospital
1650 Cedar Avenue
Montreal H3G 1A4

Ecole d'orthophonie et
 d'audiologie
Université de Montréal
2375 Côte Ste-Catherine
Montreal H3T 1A8

Sir Mortimer B. Davis Jewish
 General Hospital
Department of Audiology and
 Speech Pathology
3755 Chemin de la Côte
 Ste-Catherine
Montreal H3T 1E2

There are about a hundred centres (school boards, universities, hospitals, etc.) concerned with speech disorders in the Province of Quebec. Not all of them focus on stuttering.

Saskatchewan
Saskatchewan Speech and
 Hearing Association
79 Rawlinson Crescent
Regina S4S 6B7

Czechoslovakia

Dr F. Sram
Nad Privozern 11
1, Prague 414700

Denmark

Inspectorate of Special
 Education
(Inspectionen for Special-
 undervisningen)

Speech Handicapped Division
Vester Voldgade 117
1552 Copenhagen V.
Telephone: (01) 12-89-93

France

Hôpital neurologique de Lyon
Laboratoire de neuro-
   psychologie et de réeducation
   du langage
24 quai St Vincent
69001 Lyon

Fédération Française des
   orthophonistes
39 rue Pascal
75013 Paris

Institut des bégues
185 Boulevard President
   Wilson
33000 Bordeaux

Greece

Ministry of Health and
   Welfare
Health Protection and
   Promotion Division
17 Aristotelous Street
Athens

There are no special centres
for research and treatment of
stuttering in Greece. Treatment
is undertaken by local mental
health units. There are no
Greek stutterers' self-help
groups.

Israel

School of Communication
   Disturbances
Chim Shiba Medical Centre
Tel-Hashomer

Italy

Societa Italiana di Audiologia
   e Fonatria – SAF
Via Ticino 7
00198 Roma

Japan

The following list gives the
location of speech pathologists
in Japan who have been
certified by the American
Speech and Hearing
Association. Information
about the organizations
concerned was not available in
all cases, so in some cases
individual contacts are named.

Ministry of Health and
   Welfare
2 Kasumgaseki 1 Chome
Chiyoda-Ku
Tokyo

Sachiyuki Hamamoto
Tokyo Speech Clinic
1-17 Jingumae Shibuya
Tokyo

Dr Vchisugawa
4-12-15 Honkugenvma
Fujisawa-shi
Kanagawa-ken

Tsukuba University
1-1-1 Tennodai
Sakuramura
Niihari-gun
Ibarragi-ken

M.Q. Denny
18-13 Minami-Senju
Arakawa-Ku
Tokyo 116

C.C. Elliott
3-11-53 Minami Azabu
Minato-Ku
Tokyo 106

S.S. Ladd
c/o Deloitte, Haskins, and
  Sells
CPO Box 1193
Tokyo 100-91

C.A. Shimizu
4-12-14 Yushima
Bunkyo-Ku
Kokyo

R.J. Dunham
Nagamino Dai 2 Chome
Nada-Ku Kobe

M.L. Mason
PSC Box 2104
Yokota Ab
APO 96328SF
Yokota

Netherlands

Nederlandse Vereniging voor
  Logopedie en Foniatire
(Netherlands Association for
  Logopedics and Phoniatrics)
Oosthaven 52
2801 PE, Gouda

Stichting Institut voor
  Slechthorenden en
  Spraakgebrekkigen
(Foundation of People with
  Hearing and Speech Defects)
Jaltadaheerd 63
9737 HK Groningen

New Zealand

New Zealand Speech
  Therapists Association
1 Pere Street
Auckland 5

New Zealand Speech
  Therapists Association
Speech Therapy Clinic
George Street Normal School
Dunedin

Poland

Akademia Medyczna W.
  Pozania
60-355
Poznan

Republic of South Africa

Department of Speech
  Pathology and Audiology
University of Pretoria
Pretoria 0002

Department of Speech
  Pathology and Audiology
University of the
  Witwatersrand
Milner Park
Johannesburg 2001

Department of Speech and
  Hearing Therapy
University of Durban-Westville
Private Bag x54001
Durban 4001

Department of Logopedics
University of Cape Town
7 Dalston Road
Observatory 7925

The South African Speech and
  Hearing Association
PO Box 31782
Braamfontein 2017

Sweden

Swedish Association of
  Logopedics and Phonetics
Danderyds Sjukhus
182-88 Danderyd

Svenska Logopedforbundet
Foenatriska Avdelningen
Regionjukhuset
581-85 Linkoping

Institutionen for Logopedi och
  foenatri
vid Sahlgrenska Sjuhuset
Foenatriska Avdelningen
Goteborgs Universitet
413-45 Goteborg
Telephone: 031-60-10-00

Switzerland

International Society of
  Logopedics
Avenue de la Gare
CH-1003, Lausanne

Dr J. Sopko
34 Killmattenstrasse
CH-4105 Basel

Abteilung für Sprach- und
  Stimmstörungen der ORL-
  Klinik
Universitätsspital Zurich
Bergstrasse 94
CH-8032 Zurich

Phoniatrische Abteilung des
  Kantonsspitals Basel
Petergraben 4
CH-4000 Basel

Hör-, Stimm- und Sprach-
  abteilung der ORL-Klinik
Inselspital
CH-3010 Bern

Phoniatrie der ORL-Klinik
Kantonsspital
CH-6004 Luzern

Abteilung für Gehör-, Sprach-
  und Stimmheilkunde der
  ORL-Klinik
Kantonsspital
CH-9000 St Gallen

United Kingdom

College of Speech Therapists
6 Lechmere Road
London NW2 5BU

Stammering Research
Department of Physiology
University Medical School
Edinburgh University
Teviot Place
Edinburgh, Scotland EH8 9AG
Telephone: 031-332-3607

Centre for Personal Construct
    Psychology
132 Warwick Way
London SW1V 4JD

Department of Linguistic
    Science
University of Reading
Reading, Berkshire

Warneford Hospital
Oxford, Oxfordshire

Speech Therapy Unit
The City Literacy Institute
Keeley House
London WC2

Bloomsbury, Hampstead, and
    Islington Speech Therapy
    Services
Finsbury Health Centre
Pine Street
London EC1
Telephone: 01-278-2323
    ext. 325

People needing advice or
treatment outside London can
apply to local health centres
for appraisal and therapy
under the National Health
Service.

United States

Alabama
The Chairman
Department of Communicative
    Disorders
University of Alabama
University, Tuscaloosa 35486

Speech and Hearing Clinic
1199 Haley Center
Auburn University
Auburn 36849

Arizona
Department of Speech and
    Hearing Sciences
University of Arizona
Tucson 85721

California
Communicative Disorders
University of Southern
    California
Los Angeles 90008

Department of Speech
    Pathology (Communicative
    Disorders)
California State University
Long Beach 90840

Department of Speech and
    Hearing
University of California
Santa Barbara 93106

Florida
Speech Pathology
University of Tampa
Tampa 33606

Communicative Disorders
University of Florida
Gainesville 904

Georgia
Speech Pathology
University of Georgia
Athens 30601

Illinois
Department of Communicative
   Disorders
2299 Sheridan Road
Northwestern University
Evanston 60201

The Director
Stuttering Programs
Department of Language and
   Speech Pathology
Northwestern University
Evanston 60201

Foundation for Fluency Inc.
4801 West Peterson Avenue
Suite 218
Chicago 60646

Iowa
The Director
Department of Speech
   Pathology
University of Iowa
Iowa City 52242

Kansas
Department of Communicative
   Disorders and Sciences
PO Box 75
Wichita State University
Wichita 67208

Maryland
American Speech-Language-
   Hearing Association (ASHA)
10801 Rockville Pike
Rockville 20852
Telephone: (301) 897-5700

Massachusetts
Department of Communication
   Disorders
Boston University
48 Cummington Street
Boston 02215

Special Education Department
Boston University
Boston 02215

Michigan
National Council of the
   Stutterer
PO Box 8171
Grand Rapids 49508

The Director
Language, Speech, and
   Hearing Clinic
Department of Speech
   Pathology and Audiology
Western Michigan University
Kalamazoo 49008

Speech Pathology
Eastern Michigan University
Ypsilanti 48197

Minnesota
Department of Communication
   Disorders
115 Shevlin Hall
University of Minnesota
Minneapolis 55455

Missouri
Department of Sociology and
   Anthropology
University of Missouri
St Louis 63121

Montana
Speech and Pathology
University of Montana
Missoula 59801
Telephone: (406) 243-0211

New Hampshire
Speech and Pathology
University of New Hampshire
Durham 03824
Telephone: (603) 868-5511

New York
The John Jay College
City University of New York
444 West 56th Street
New York 10019

Behavioral Sciences
Cornell University Medical
   College
925 East 68th Street
New York 10021

Department of Speech
Brooklyn College
City University of New York
Brooklyn 11210

Hofstra University Speech and
   Hearing Center
Hempstead 11551

Speech Department
Karen Horney Clinic
New York 10001

North Dakota
Speech, Language, and
   Hearing Clinic
PO Box 8040 University Station
Grand Forks 58202
Telephone: (701) 777-3232

Ohio
Speech Pathology
Bowling Green State University
Bowling Green 43402
Telephone: (419) 353-8411

Pennsylvania
Department of Speech
   Pathology
University of Pittsburgh
Pittsburgh 15260

Speech Pathology
Temple University
Philadelphia 19104

Tennessee
Stadium and Yale Hearing and
   Speech Center
Knoxville 37916

Texas
School of Communication
   Disorders
Central Campus
University of Houston
Houston 77004

Stuttering Center
Baylor College
Houston 77004

Utah
Department of Speech
  Pathology and Audiology
University of Utah
1201 Behavioral Science
  Building
Salt Lake City 84112

Virginia
Division for Children with
  Communication Disorders
The Council for Exceptional
  Children
1920 Association Drive
Reston 22091
Telephone: (703) 620-3660

Department of Psychology
Hollins Communications
  Research Institute
Hollins College
Roanoke 24020

Washington
Department of Speech and
  Hearing Sciences
Eagleton Hall
University of Washington
Seattle 98195

Department of Speech
Washington State University
Pullman 99163

Washington DC
The Speech Foundation of
  America
5139 Klingle Street
20307

Army Audiology and Speech
  Center
Walter Reed Army Medical
  Center
20307

Wisconsin
Speech Pathology
Marquette University
Milwaukee 53233
Telephone: (414) 344-1000

USSR

Professor S. Taptapova
Vspolniiperd 16 K 2 KV 86
Moscou K1

West Germany

Bundeszentrale für gesund-
  heitliche Aufklärung
Ostmerheimerstrasse 200
D-5000 Köln 91
Postfach 91 01 52

Klinik für Kommunikations-
  störungen
Langenbeckstrasse
Mainz

Deutsche Gesellschaft für
  Sprachheilkunde e.v.
Rostocker Strasse 62
2000 Hamburg 1

Zentralverband für Logopadie
Goethestr. 9
5000 Köln 41
Telephone: 02234179651

Index